FOLK
MEDICINE
IN
AMERICA
TODAY

FOLK MEDICINE IN AMERICA TODAY

JOHN
HEINERMAN, PH.D.

Twin Streams
KENSINGTON PUBLISHING CORP.
www.kensingtonbooks.com

TWIN STREAMS BOOKS are published by

Kensington Publishing Corp.
850 Third Avenue
New York, NY 10022

All Kensington titles, imprints and distributed lines are available at special quantity discounts for bulk purchases for sales promotion, premiums, fund-raising, educational or institutional use.

Special book excerpts or customized printings can also be created to fit specific needs. For details, write or phone the office of the Kensington Special Sales Manager: Kensington Publishing Corp., 850 Third Avenue, New York, NY 10022. Attn. Special Sales Department. Phone: 1-800-221-2647.

Twin Streams and the TS logo Reg. U.S. Pat. & TM Off.

ISBN 0-7582-0050-1

First Kensington Trade Paperback Printing: October, 2001
10 9 8 7 6 5 4 3 2 1

Printed in the United States of America

To Doña Ascensión Solórsano,
the last of her kind, and a truly remarkable folk healer.

This woman was the last member of the long-since-extinct San Juan Indian tribe of California. Her mother (who died at 84) and her father (who passed on at 82) were both full-blood Indians and spoke the language of their tribe all their lives. Doña learned it from them, but it had scarcely been spoken since 1850. The parents also taught their daughter much about what was by then a relatively dead Indian culture, with those three being the last survivors of a once thriving and vigorous tribe.

For many decades in adult life, this incredible woman was widely recognized and highly respected as one of the very best practitioners of *curanderismo* to have ever lived in "The Golden State." "Her little home in Gilroy, California, was a free hospital for down-and-outs of every nationality and creed. And here the sick and ailing were treated with Indian and Spanish herb medicines and were seen through to the last with motherly care and no thought of recompense."*

During much of 1929 and the early part of January 1930, this noble Native-American woman very patiently and willingly shared the bulk of her medical and cultural knowledge with Smithnonian ethnologist John P. Harrington at Monterey, California, in spite of the fact that she was extremely aged and very ill at the time. "So sick that she was scarcely able to sit up even at the beginning of the work, Mr. Harrington continued this work at her bedside . . . and no Indian ever showed greater fortitude than this poor soul who served the bureau up to almost her last day."*

"In spite of her age and infirmities, Doña Ascensión's mind remained remarkably clear and her memory was exceptional. No greater piece of good fortune has ever attended ethnological research of a tribe that was culturally of the greatest importance, forming an all but lost link between the [Native American] cultures of northern and southern California."*

*From the *Forty-Seventh Annual Report of the Bureau of American Ethnology to the Smithsonian Institution 1929–1930* (Washington, D.C.: United States Government Printing Office, 1932; pp. 3–5).

Contents

HOW I BECAME INVOLVED WITH FOLK MEDICINE

My father's mother was of Magyar descent. These are the dominant people of Hungary, whence my grandmother and her German husband came. The Magyars, like the Finns, whom they're related to linguistically, were a nomadic nation that migrated first (in about A.D. 460) from the Urals to the northern Caucasus and then westward some four centuries later across southern Russia into what is now Hungary and part of Rumania.

These were a people with a strong tradition of folk medicine. Their contact with the Turkish peoples expanded their botanical repertoire considerably. Their materia medica was further enhanced over time by their somewhat brief association with the Russians. When the Austro-Hungarian monarchy was established in 1867 and continued until World War I broke out, the rigid Austrian medical system sort of codified and somewhat legitimized the rural folk medicine that had been haphazardly practiced by the Magyars for a number of centuries.

In those times it wasn't uncommon for peasants to refer not only to their family lineages, but also to the individual tribes or bands to which they belonged. Certain skills such as blacksmithing, wood carving, barbering, and shoemaking were often passed down from father to son over successive generations. The same thing held true for folk healing, which, at that time, was primarily entrusted to women.

Grandmother Barbara Liebhardt Kaplan Heinerman was one of those who, typically speaking, "came up through the ranks"—she was an eighth- or ninth-generation herbalist and acquired her healing skills in several different ways. One of these was through close observation and study, which came by working with her mother and still-living grandmother while a young girl whenever they rendered natural treatments to the sick in need. Another, even more profound, way was by *inheriting* from both of them a certain *knack* for healing, something that I've dubbed "a healing intuition."

This peculiar "gift," for so it can be rightfully called, skipped my father and brother but, for reasons still unknown even to this day, settled in me at a very early age. I clearly remember the first time I felt it stirring within me. I was in the sixth grade attending Maeser Elementary School in Provo, Utah, where my family then resided. One day at school in the lunchroom, one of my chums complained to several of the boys around him including me of having a gut ache. He moaned and groaned something fierce and kept holding his stomach and sides with his hands in hopes of making the pains somehow disappear.

As I look back on the incident now, I'm convinced that what the kid probably suffered from was just a bad case of intestinal gas. He no doubt got it from bolting his food down. (Have you ever known a kid to carefully chew what he eats?) Almost instinctively I knew what to do, though I couldn't say *why* the remedy worked—I just *knew* that it would! I went over to one of the lunch ladies and asked her if she would be so kind as to warm up a glass of milk for our buddy and stir in a level teaspoon of powdered cinnamon, which they dutifully did. After drinking this concoction and waiting for several minutes, our little friend pronounced himself over his self-induced gastrointestinal torment. This was my very first episode of "healing intuition," but there would be some others to follow as I matured to manhood. The kids started calling me "Doc" after that, and the nickname pretty well stuck all through high school and even into college somewhat.

Folk medicine was *always* practiced in some way in my family during the whole time I was growing up. My parents never believed in having their two sons get any kind of immunizations and I was thankfully spared from having my body poisoned and immune system compromised at a very early age, as most other children are unfortunately subject to while still very young. Whenever my brother Joseph or I would get sick, we were always given warm herbal teas, citrus juices (for their vitamin C content), and an oily extract from the *Oleum percamorphum* fish, once obtainable from most local pharmacies (and which fulfilled our bodies' vitamin A requirements very nicely).

On other occasions, we would be "administered" to by my father and another church elder, both of whom held the "higher priesthood," which presumably let them conduct such an ordinance in an official capacity. It's all part of a rather novel Mormon healing ritual involving "consecrated oil"—virgin olive oil that has been "blessed" by church elders—and the "laying on of hands." With the necessary childlike faith to make it work, my brother and I usually got well within a very short time. This ritual is still practiced among the Mormons today to some extent, yet because of a lack of faith and trust in God, very, very few actual miracles of recovery ever happen anymore.

My brother and I were both born at home and delivered by my father and Grandmother Barbara. We were raised on whole cow's milk and lots of fresh fruits and vegetables and whole grains. We were taught early on to avoid candy and all types of sweets, being told that they were all "very poisonous" to the system and could make us very sick if we ingested them. The dramatic comparison of a spoonful of white sugar and an equivalent amount of rat poison was indelibly etched in our young memories, never to be forgotten. This singular instruction, while obviously preserving our health through life, created quite a stir among our school friends, who thought we both were just "plain nuts" for refusing to eat anything sweet, including candy, cookies, cake, and even ice cream.

I remember this one time while I was in the fourth grade at Maeser School when my teacher, Mrs. Babcock, who died some years later of diabetes, hauled me down to the principal's office for wasting what she called "good food" by throwing in the classroom trash can some Valentine's Day cookies that I and others had been given. Needless to say, the principal didn't act on her complaint, but my brother and I soon developed an unpleasant reputation for being "crazy" and having equally "nutty" parents to boot.

Sometimes when I suffered more serious health problems, such as my strange attack of gallstones at age six or a right-side groin hernia at age twelve, I would be treated with some of Grandmother Barbara's "tried-and-true" remedies. My gallstones were eliminated by my drinking of plenty of warm potato peeling broth, and my hernia was treated with daily swallows of slippery elm tea while a truss held the hernia in until nature herself could repair the small tear in my muscle tissue.

My brother and I were always taught by our parents and grandmothers that "doctors can't be trusted" and that "medical science (for the most part) is wrong and inspired by the Evil One." So forcefully were these ideas ingrained in our young minds that even when we became full-grown adults and college-educated, with minds of our own to think as we damn well pleased, they still were firmly fixed. In 1974 while I was returning from a business trip to Idaho Falls, Idaho, the right rear tire on my Chevy pickup truck came off on the freeway near Malad, causing the vehicle to suddenly swerve around to the right in a counterclockwise fashion and flip over twice before coming to a rest in the opposite lane of traffic.

A beveled rearview mirror attached to my windshield struck my skull with enough force to inflict a serious wound. But I remained conscious through the whole ordeal, though I lost a great deal of blood in the process. When the ambulance came to rush me to the hospital, I refused to let the attendants do so. The county sheriff on the scene, thinking I was delusional because of the accident, intended to handcuff me to the stretcher so they could do their job with less fuss, whereupon I verbally threatened him in no uncertain terms that if he attempted to do so, I would hire the meanest, nastiest lawyer in those parts and sue him for all he was worth, and bring ruin and shame to him for the rest of his life. Sensing that I wasn't bluffing at all, he backed away and muttered something to the effect that I could die for all he cared.

I permitted the paramedics to at least bandage up the wound the best they could and transport me to the home of the nearest Mormon bishop in that little hamlet. I asked Bishop Jones if he and his counselors (whom he telephoned to come over to his place) would "administer" to me. They did and I had just enough faith to feel the bleeding stop and my severe headache disappear almost instantaneously. I then called a friend of mine in Idaho Falls, one Dee Mar Brower, who came down in his vehicle in about an hour and took me back to his home.

Once at Dee's home, I instructed Dee and his wife as to what they should do. Both were totally unacquainted with something of such a severe nature as this. In fact, Dee's wife, Regina, almost fainted away after removing the bloody bandages and seeing just how deep the wound penetration was. But with some salt and whiskey they thoroughly cleansed out the wound and put a new dressing of bandages on. I remained in their care for about a week before I was sufficiently well again to travel back to Utah on my own. Seeing as how they knew virtually nothing about herbs, vitamins, or minerals, I kept the things we used very simple: some cayenne pepper, powdered turmeric, table salt, cheap Southern Comfort whiskey for external use, and lots of citrus juices, cooked oatmeal, and cooked animal protein (particularly fried and baked liver with onions) for the internal nourishment. Needless to say I fully recovered in about six weeks and *without* the benefit of a single medical doctor! (Of course, I *wouldn't* recommend that the average person ever attempt such a thing if placed in a similar situation. I relate this for anecdotal purposes only.)

These, then, are some of the facts concerning my gradual involvement with folk medicine from childhood up. The journey has been interesting, though sometimes fraught with heartache and disappointment. But such a life-long trip has its own rewards, especially when someone of my particularly divinely endowed talents is able to help others in some special way and see them restored to health again sans the torture routinely inflicted by the medical profession.

But I will be the first to admit that folk medicine may, in fact, not be for everyone. A case in point: Back in the early 1980s I accompanied a small group of medical graduates from the Oregon Naturopathic School on a cross-country healing journey of sorts. I was along more for the ride and to do a series of write-ups on the whole affair for a monthly newsletter I then edited (*The Herb Report*) than as a teacher.

Somewhere in our travels, at one of the many rest stops dotting our nation's highways, we came upon a small crowd of people gathered around a young boy of about ten years of age lying upon the grass. He was in the throes of a grand mal seizure. And judging from the hysterical behavior of his very distraught mother and extremely anxious father, it was probably the first one he'd ever had. Someone had had the good sense to place a small stick between the kid's jaws early on so he wouldn't end up biting his tongue to pieces.

Responding to the pleas of the desperate mom for someone to help them, one of our group stepped forward and offered my services without even bothering to ask me first just how I felt about the matter. Hearing that I was an accomplished folk healer of sorts, they virtually demanded that I do something. I quickly surveyed the situation, pondered it over in my heart for a moment, then politely declined and walked away. The naturopathic students followed close on my heels, visibly annoyed by my refusal to participate and ostracizing me for my decision.

In response to one sharply worded question of "You knew what to do, didn't you?" I turned around and replied that I did. But then I gave my logical reason for denying the parents my assistance. I explained that I would have had to ask them to permit me, a total stranger, to remove their son's trousers and shorts, spread his legs apart, and, while pushing his scrotum to one side, apply strong pressure with the fingertips of my right hand against a particular nerve for a minute or so to bring the kid out of his epileptic attack.

"Do you think for a moment that in their condition of hysteria they would have been mentally fit to grant such a shocking request to someone like myself traveling in the company of a bunch of other guys? Gentlemen, I don't know about any of you, but I want to finish this trip with my freedom intact and not sitting in a lousy jail somewhere on trumped up charges of presumed child abuse!" And that ended the discussion right there, followed by a few mumbled apologies before we resumed our journey.

The art of folk medicine is a life's worth of cultural acquisition in which many things are slowly learned, carefully tested, and thought-fully remembered for future use somewhere. Unlike knowledge that can be quickly gleaned, this isn't something obtained in the "fast track" of life, but rather studiously cultivated in an environment of caring compassion with faith, humility, and if one's lucky enough, "a healing intuition" of some kind to go with the rest of it.

Chapter One

FOLK MEDICINE IN ANCIENT TIMES

(Egypt, Greece, India, and China)

A Matter of Semantics

Social scientists who study other cultures have often had a difficult time quantifying some of the aspects of the various indigenous peoples they're investigating. The term "folk medicine" is one of these. In the beginning it was simple enough (or so they thought) to use terms such as "primitive," "traditional," and "non-Western" in discussing the medicine of the *common* people and "scientific," "modern," and "Western" to describe the more advanced care of the presumably "enlightened" societies.

Early ethnologists and anthropologists spoke and wrote unabashedly about "primitive medicine" as consisting "primarily of magico-religious factors, utilizing just a few rational elements," as Erwin Ackerknect, among others, was prone to do in the early 1940s. But following World War II, studies of peasant communities became fashionable, and social scientists began discovering, to their delight and amazement, that such peoples actually possessed a "folk culture" of some type. Not surprisingly then their medical systems usually were referred to as "folk medicine."

"Natural" Medicine of the Common Folk

Thus was born the term that not only forms the lead title of this book, but is mentioned quite frequently throughout the text. Yet if the truth be fully known, "folk medicine" is actually more "natural medicine" in the full sense of the word. Embodied within the cultural parameters of this "natural" medicine is the "supernatural"—one works along more conventional lines, such as food choices, remedial treatments, temperature changes, strong winds, blood or air "trapped in the body," and mood shifts, while the other clearly operates in a realm all its own, usually consisting of invisible deities, spirits, ghosts, and other nonmaterial entities, and is almost wholly dependent upon the factor of faith to make such things possible for the living.

"Natural medicine" typically embraces a wide range of services and healing modalities, which can include but are not limited to naturopathy, chiropractic, acupuncture, reflexology, massage, herbal remedies, aromatherapy, and thalassotherapy. This system of medicine also tends to explain illness in impersonal, systemic terms; sensate agents play no role.

In naturalistic or folk systems of healing, health always conforms to an equilibrium model: When the basic body elements—the "humors," the yin and yang, and the Ayurvedic *dosha*—are in the balance appropriate to the age and condition of the individual, health results. When this balance is upset for any reason, either from within or from without, by natural forces such as heat, cold, or occasionally strong emotions, illness invariably follows. Although the equilibrium principle in such folk or naturalistic systems is expressed in a number of ways, contemporary descriptions reveal the primary role of heat and cold as the principle threats to health.

Words such as these sometimes refer to actual temperature, but more often they tend to describe qualities not directly related to heat or cold. In the Hispanic folk medicine of the American Southwest and all of Latin America, for instance, foods, medicinal herbs, and many other substances, conditions, and events (such as ice, menstruation and pregnancy, and an eclipse of the moon) are classified as hot, cold, or neutral in the sense of innate qualities. The conceptual principle is similar to that used in the United States in "hard" and "soft" water, "hard" and "soft" beverages, and "dry" and "sweet" wines. Common sense tells us that liquids aren't hard, soft, or dry in the usual sense of the words, and a social scientist from Mars would certainly be puzzled by our queer terminology.

Contemporary folk or naturalistic systems of healing resemble each other in an important historical sense: The bulk of their explanations and practices represent simplified and popularized legacies from the "Great Tradition" medicine of ancient classical civilizations, particularly those of Egypt, Greece, India, and China. Unlike personalistic systems, known largely through modern anthropological studies, folk medical systems are shown by historical records to reach way back into the distant past, even as far back as some 4,000 years ago. A knowledge of the origin and development of these systems enables us to understand the many modern variants that there are to folk medicine in general worldwide.

Ancient Egyptian Medicine

Some insight into the medical practice of ancient Egypt may be derived from human remains, from representations of bodies showing signs of disease, and from occasional references to disease in the nonmedical papyri and stelae of that particular civilization. However, by far the most important sources of our knowledge are the medical papyri themselves. According to Clement of Alexandria, writing in the second century A.D., the forty-two books of human knowledge possessed by the ancient Egyptians included six of medical content:

37. The structure of the human body
38. Diseases in general
39. The instruments of the doctors
40. Treatment remedies
41. The eyes and their diseases
42. Diseases of women

Ancient Egyptian medicine is best reflected in the surviving medical papyri that were found in the last century or in the early years of the twentieth century. These are listed in Table 1.1.

TABLE 1.1. THE MOST IMPORTANT MEDICAL PAPYRI

Title	Location	Approx. Date of Copy	Contents
Edwin Smith	New York	1550 B.C.	Surgical, mainly trauma
Ebers	Leipzig	1500 B.C.	General, mainly medical
Kahun	University College, London	1820 B.C.	Gynecological
Hearst	California	1450 B.C.	General medical
Chester Beatty VI	British Museum (10686), London	1200 B.C.	Rectal diseases
Berlin	Berlin	1200 B.C.	General medical
London	British Museum (10059)	1300 B.C.	Mainly magical
Carlsberg VIII	Copenhagen	1300 B.C.	Gynecological
Ramesseum II, IV, V	Oxford	1700 B.C.	Gynecological, ophthalmic, and pediatric
London and Leiden	British Museum (10072) and Leiden	A.D. 250	General medical and magical
Crocodilopolis	Vienna	A.D. 150	General
Brooklyn snake	Brooklyn	300 B.C.	Snake bite

In most cases the foregoing medical papyri were offered for sale with little or no detail of their provenance whatsoever. It seems plausible that some at least came from the tomb of doctors, but in no case is it possible to link a medical papyrus with a known doctor of the time. They are written on papyrus and, with the single exception of that of Ramesseum V, in hieratic style. The writing is horizontal from right to left, except in the fragments of Ramesseum III, IV, and V, in which it is in vertical columns (a common practice in the Middle Kingdom period).

Although there is considerable repetition in some of the papyri, there is good reason to believe that we possess only a small fraction of the medical papyri, so many of which must have been lost due to the ravages of time. Many papyri would certainly have been destroyed during tomb robbing, some were used as fuel, and a number were actually used to prepare magical remedies. Paragraph 262 of the Ebers papyrus, also called Ebers 262, itself describes the use of "an old book cooked in oil (or grease)" as a local application to the belly to help a child pass urine. A medical text might have been considered particularly effective.

A comparison of the two most famous Egyptian papyri—the Edwin Smith surgical papyrus and the Ebers papyrus, which were of about the same period and believed to have been taken from the same tomb—will show that there existed some 3,500 years ago two systems of medicine, working side by side, serving both the interests of the hierarchy as well as those of the common people. The contents of the Edwin Smith papyrus are divided into seventeen pages describing forty-eight cases, nearly all the victims of some kind of trauma. It differs from most of the other medical papyri in its definite and logical approach, being an "instruction" book rather than simply a compilation of remedies, or "remedy book." This enables scholars to visualize the ancient Egyptian doctor's examination of the patient, and they can gain considerable insight into the processes by which he arrived at a diagnosis. This contrasts with much of the Ebers papyrus, which usually assumes that the diagnosis has already been made and then follows with a remedy to eliminate the named disease. This is usually given without any indication of the symptoms of the disease, and in many instances, it is now impossible for anyone to know what was the actual disease involved.

The Edwin Smith papyrus has an instant appeal to the doctor of today. It contains much that relates to current surgical practice and it isn't too difficult to see the workings of the pharonic doctor. One can easily visualize him examining his patient and can read his mind as he reaches a diagnosis, and a scholar can identify with him in his treatment of the patient. In keeping with the pragmatic approach, it is remarkably free of magic.

Not so, however, with the Ebers papyrus. The Ebers is a compendium of many different original sources assembled in an order that often appears random. There are some eleven spells in addition to the three basic spells in the first three paragraphs of the papyrus. It shares this distinction of "folk magic" with a number of other medical papyri, particularly the Hearst, Berlin, and London.

While Edwin Smith is highly organized and logically presented, the Ebers of about the same period is not. Its rather haphazard order more strongly suggests the input of folk healers, instead of physicians or surgeons, as the former does. It wanders all over the place, going from a skin rash remedy—milk and pure oil mixed together and applied freely—to a crocodile bite treatment, before jumping to cough remedies and certain eye diseases. But it is the frequent reference to the supernatural or magic that clearly indicates it to have been a popular medical text for common folks like you and me. Paragraphs 242 through 247, for instance, speak of remedies reputed to have been prepared by certain Egyptian gods for their own use or sometimes prepared by one god for use by another, as paragraph 247 seems to suggest: "A sixth remedy which Isis made for Ra himself to eliminate the disease that is in his head."

Another clear difference between Edwin Smith and Ebers is what each covers and *doesn't* cover in terms of anatomy. The former offers quite a remarkable insight into an anatomical knowledge of the skull and chest (where it suddenly stops), which would probably make it comparable to any modern surgical text for those regions of the upper body. Ebers, on the other hand, pays a great amount of attention to the large bowel, rectum, and anus in terms of things that can be done to soothe, heal, and help them work more efficiently. The numerous remedies given are intended to "settle," "cool or refresh," and "drive out heat" from these different parts of the gastrointestinal tract. Both the language style and remedy descriptions are more indicative of native folk healers working along natural principles than of surgeons prone to operating, setting fractures, and mending broken limbs.

It is clear that some 3,500 years ago, conventional medicine (as reflected in the Smith papyrus) and folk medicine (as exemplified in Ebers) peacefully coexisted and worked together for the common good of everyone. But just like today, the better educated and more affluent gravitated to the surgeons and their drugs, while the less learned and poorer classes settled for folk healers.

A common phrase shared in both medical texts is "placing the hand," which seems to have been a hallmark of all Egyptian practitioners, the way carrying a stethoscope is today. For regular physicians, this was probably more to establish a diagnosis of some kind, whereas for folk healers it may have been intended as a cure, as in the "laying on of hands."

Egyptian doctors, both conventional and unorthodox, were held in high esteem by neighboring countries. In response to a request, Ramses II dispatched a doctor, known from Akkadian texts as Parianmakhu, to the Hittite court "to prepare herbs for Karunta, King of the land of Tarhuntas." He also added as an afterthought that if further medical help was needed, he could send along his "personal court surgeon" at a later date.

The ancient Egyptian pharmacopoeia contained a wide range of animal products. Sometimes there was a sound pharmacological basis for the benefit that was expected. In other cases, the substance simply provided a convenient vehicle for other constituents. In certain cases the remedy was based on the characteristics of the donor animal, which were deemed desirable.

Few medicaments had wider use in ancient Egypt than honey. Honey was used both externally and internally in hundreds of the remedies in the medical papyri. It was used partly as a vehicle and partly for its own intrinsic properties when applied externally or taken internally. Honey is largely composed of sugars (mainly lucose and fructose), and was of particular value in a society where the sugar beet and cane sugar were unknown. Its sweetness was clearly intended as a linctus to relieve cough in Ebers. It has powerful antibacterial and antifungal properties, which are due mainly to the osmotic effect of the high concentrations of sugar.

Much interest has centered on honey's use on open wounds. The osmotic effect reduces swelling, but more importantly, bacteria do not grow in honey. Honey has been demonstrated to accelerate wound healing, and similar benefits follow its use on burns and ulcers. Internal use in children with gastroenteritis shortened the duration of diarrhea. Its use on open wounds appears to have been fully justified. In fact, the therapeutic potential of honey is grossly underestimated at present by the medical profession.

Milk also had extensive use, often as a convenient vehicle, a role that is indicated by the failure to specify the proportion in a mixture. The following is a remedy for an obstruction of the stomach, as found in the Ebers papyrus:

> *tiam* (unknown plant), 1/16; grains from umbrella pine of Byblos (*peret-sheny*), 1/16; valerian (*shasha*), 1/8; cyperus grass of the island 1/16; cyperus grass of the garden (*gyw n hesep*), 1/16; wine and milk; to be eaten and swallowed with sweet beer, to make him well immediately.

It seems likely that the wine and milk are included merely as a vehicle to make the other ingredients easier to take. The origin of the milk is unspecified, but on other occasions it is indicated as the cow, ass, or even "human." Remedies containing milk were most commonly taken by mouth but also as an enema, to be poured into the vagina, or applied to the eyes, the ears (as curds), or even the skin; most of these milk applications are found in Ebers.

Animal fats had an extensive use in the prescriptions of ancient Egypt, partly because of their ability to make a greasy ointment and partly in the hope of transferring some desirable characteristic of the animal. Perhaps the most remarkable example comes from Ebers 465:

> Another [remedy] to cause hair to grow on a bald person: fat of lion, 1; fat of hippopotamus, 1; fat of crocodile, 1; fat of cat, 1; fat of snake, 1; fat of ibex, 1; make as one thing, smear (or anoint) the head of the bald person with it.

It is interesting to contemplate the cost of this remedy and the powerful element of suggestion that would accompany its use. However, in this case there is no comment on efficacy, which sometimes took such forms as "really effective—a million times!" Other species used included the antelope, ass, fish, goose, ostrich, ox, mouse, and sheep. Preparations including animal fat could be taken internally or as an enema but were most frequently used as an external application.

Fresh meat was widely prescribed for application to a wound on the first day. This recalls the common folk remedy of applying a beef steak to a black eye. Meat can provide blood-clotting factors, and pioneer neurosurgeons used fresh pigeon and chicken breast meat to control oozing.

The prescription of meat to be taken by mouth may be an example of dietary treatment. An obscure section of the Ebers papyrus (284–293) comprises remedies to cause the heart to receive bread. It is likely that "bread" refers to food in general, and the distinction between the heart (*ib*) and the stomach—literally the "mouth of the heart" (*r-ib*)—is often uncertain. This group of prescriptions abounds with nutritious items, and three include "fat meat."

Of all the animal products, the most valued by the ancient Egyptian doctors was liver, which contains 90 percent of the body store of vitamin B_{12}, essential for the prevention of megaloblastic (pernicious) anemia. Raw liver by mouth and later injection of liver extract were the basis of therapy for megaloblastic anemia before the discovery of vitamin B_{12}. Although the Ebers papyrus periodically makes reference to liver, it isn't clear whether or not it is for something like this.

The second major therapeutic implication is deficiency of vitamin A causing night blindness, which can be treated by eating liver, a rich source of vitamin A. There is one instance of the ingestion of raw liver being recommended for "a woman who cannot see," and one of the local application of cooked liver for a case of *sharu*-blindness. Both texts suggest that liver is a logical solution for failing sight or for treating night blindness. In Ebers 267 is a recommendation for the oral administration of ox liver (not specified to be raw) for "accumulations" (*henau*) in the urine.

Some drugs of mineral origin were employed as well, the two most common being natron (*hesmen*) and ordinary salt (*wadju*). Natron was deposited as a mixture of evaporites in areas that had previously been flooded, and subsequently evaporated to dryness as a result of climatic changes. The material was freely available and used extensively in mummification. The composition of natron varied greatly from one location to another, but the major constituents were sodium chloride, sodium sulphate, sodium carbonate, and sodium bicarbonate. Its use in the solid state or as a paste had a powerful osmotic effect, drawing out fluid and reducing swelling. This was a role similar to that of the European Glauber's salts, which were pure sodium sulphate. Natron was generally alkaline, depending on the proportion of sodium carbonate.

Natron's most extensive use was as an external application, often under a bandage. Perhaps the clearest and most logical use is in Hearst 140 with a similar recipe in Ebers 557:

> Another remedy to draw (bring) pus (*ryt*); *ipshenen* (unknown), 1; natron, 1; clay (or gypsum) from the potter's kiln, 1; carob, 1; terebinth resin, 1; bring flour of date (*nyt net benri*); make as one thing and bandage with it.

Ignoring the other components, natron would be appropriate for superficial sepsis. Ebers 595 also prescribes natron for drawing out pus. It was sometimes prescribed along with common salt.

Salt was often specified as the salt of Lower Egypt, where perhaps it was obtained by the evaporation of sea water. Its main effect at high concentrations is osmotic, as is natron's, but in a solution of approximately 1 percent, its osmotic pressure is close to that of body fluids. Warm salt solutions are mildly emetic. Salt was often included in prescriptions with many components and perhaps was added mainly for its taste. It had a very wide use, being taken by mouth, by enema, as an anal suppository for hemorrhoids, and as a local application to the eyes, ears, and especially to the skin, where it was often held in place by a bandage.

Ancient Egyptian doctors and folk healers made extensive use of herbs and other plants. They lived in an environment that supported a wide range of indigenous plants, but they also imported certain species from countries such as Lebanon. A great number of plant species appear by their Egyptian names in the medical papyri.

Some of the more popular drugs of vegetable origin are given in Table 1.2, together with their Egyptian and scientific names. Their individual uses in pharaonic remedies are mentioned as well.

TABLE 1.2. BOTANICAL REMEDIES OF THE PHARAONIC PERIOD

Common Name	Egyptian Name	Scientific Name	Medicinal Application
asafoetida	gesfen	*Ferula foetida*	cough, diarrhea, accumulated mucus, constipation, spasms
aniseed	inset	*Pimpinella anisum*	digestion, nausea, insomnia, intestinal gas
carob	djaret	*Ceratonia siliqua*	diarrhea, worms, eye/skin inflammation, open wounds, sores, burns, body odor
celery	matet	*Apium graveolens*	demonic possession, uterine inflammation, burns, cavities
cinnamon	ti-shepses	*Cinnamonium zeylanicum*	body odor, upset stomach, gum disease, hemorrhoids
coriander	shaw	*Coriander sativum*	stomach ailments, bloody stool, illness related to magical spell casting, broken bones, fractures, insomnia, skin sores, snake bite poison
cucumber (see melon)			
cumin	tepnen	*Cuminum cymimum*	stomach problems, chest ailments, cough, mouth/tongue sores, headache, body pain
date	beneret	*Phoenix dactylifera*	swelling, leg pains, sneezing, baldness, constipation, heart problems, sickness due to magical spell casting
dill	imset	*Anethum graveolens*	body pain, headache, bad breath, gas, colic, hiccups, mummy tomb odor
fenugreek	imset	*Trigonella foenum-graecum*	eye ailments, blurred vision, indigestion, obesity, snake bite
fig	dab	*Ficus carica*	cancer, constipation, indigestion, heart problems, lung disorders, demon-induced angina or cardiac attack, hemorrhoids, skin rash
fir	ash	*Abies cilicica*	difficult birth, stiff limbs/joints, edema, swelling, worms, wounds, baldness

TABLE 1.2. BOTANICAL REMEDIES OF THE PHARAONIC PERIOD (cont.)

Common Name	Egyptian Name	Scientific Name	Medicinal Application
flaxseed	mehy	*Linum usitatissimum*	abdominal swelling, hemorrhoids, crushed fingers/toes, body pain, skin eruptions, wounds
garlic	kheten	*Allium sativum*	burns, dog bites, snake bites, bruises, worms, toothache, earache, hoarseness, epidemics, infection
grape	iareret	*Vitis vinifera*	cancer, infection, fatigue, blood impurities
juniper	wan	*Juniperus phoenicea*	flatulence, indigestion, constipation, tapeworm, asthma, headache, incense to dispel air sickness and corpse odor during mummification
leek	iaquet	*Allium kurrat*	colds, flu, bronchitis, asthma, warts, night blindness
lettuce	afet/afay	*Lactuca virosa*	swollen eyes/eyelids, abdominal pain, intestinal parasites, infection, ear infection, cough, nervousness, insomnia
lotus	seshen	*Nymphaea lotus*	liver disorders, demonic constipation, fever, nervousness, headache
melon (cucumber)	shespet	*Cucumis melo*	animal bites, fever, gum inflammation, sore tongue, sunburn, bladder problems
myrtle	khet-des	*Myrtus communis*	neuralgia, air fumigation, urinary disorders, mucus accumulation, heartburn, swelling, joint/limb stiffness, cough, skin afflictions, breathing difficulties
onion	hedju	*Allium cepa*	burns, excessive menstruation, ear problems, snake bites, cough, colds, stomach ailments
pea	tehu/peret-tehu	*Pisum sativum*	tumor, wounds, sores, fingernail or toenail fungus, burns, vaginal bleeding, mental suffering due to demonic affliction

TABLE 1.2. BOTANICAL REMEDIES OF THE PHARAONIC PERIOD (cont.)

Common Name	Egyptian Name	Scientific Name	Medicinal Application
pomegranate	inhemen	*Punica granatum*	tapeworm, plague fever, cysts, dysentery, diarrhea, stomachache, roundworm, burns, swelling, skin ailments, constipation
pyrethrum	shames	*Anacyclus pyrethrum*	skin afflictions, dandruff, head lice, nail/skin fungus
raisin	wenshi	*Vitis vinifera*	anemia, fatigue, fever
senna	gengenet	*Cassia acutifolia*	chronic constipation (not to be used when hemorrhoids are present or the stomach is inflamed)
tamarisk	iser	*Tamarix nilotica*	eye disorders, hemorrhaging, dysentery, inflammation due to evil incantations, leprosy, leg ulcers, sores, excessive menstruation
valerian	shasha	*Valeriana officinalis*	spasms, nervousness, headache, hysteria, pinworms, pimples
watermelon	bededu-ka	*Citrullus lanatus*	nervous trembling, constipation, childbirth, edema
willow	tjeret	*Salix safsaf*	poor appetite, swelling, inflammation, headache, toothache, sunburn, blisters, skin diseases
wormwood	sam	*Artemisia absinthium*	indigestion, poor appetite, worms, smashed hand/fingers/toes, bruises, cough, breathing difficulties, fever

Folk Medical Theories of the Ancient Greeks

Ancient Greek doctors and folk healers viewed the causations of all diseases from the concept of bodily "humors." This humoral pathology, as it has come to be known, is rooted in the ancient theory, first conceived by the Greeks and later passed on to other parts of the world, of nature's four essential elements for the sustenance of life: earth, water, air, and fire. By the time Hippocrates (born around 460 B.C.) came along, this theory had been augmented by the parallel concept of four qualities—hot, cold, dry, moist—which, when integrated with the original theory, produced the idea of the four "humors" with their associated qualities. These were as follows: *blood* (hot and moist), *phlegm* (cold and moist), *black bile,* also called "melancholy" (cold and dry), and *yellow bile,* or "choler" (hot and dry).

That the equilibrium theory of health was well developed in ancient Greek medicine and folk healing is evidenced by some of the Hippocratic medical writings regarding disease: "The human body contains blood, phlegm, yellow bile and black bile. These are things that make up its constitution and cause its pains and health. Health is primarily that state in which these constituent substances are in the correct proportion to each other, both in strength and quality, and are well mixed. Pain occurs when one of the substances presents either a deficiency or an excess, or is separated in the body some way and not mixed in with the others."

These four humors, wrote the acknowledged father of modern medicine, "have specific and different names because there are essential differences in their appearance. . . . They are dissimilar in their qualities of heat, cold, dryness, and moisture." Although Hippocrates appears to specify precisely in no place the qualities of the humors, he clearly comprehended these qualities and noted that they varied in quantity over the year, depending on climate and weather. Phlegm increases in the winter, he wrote, because as the coldest humor, it is most in keeping with the winter. During the spring the quantity of blood increases, stimulated by the wet and warm days of the rainy season. Because it is moist and hot, this part of the year is most in keeping with the blood. During the summer, although blood remains strong, the bile gradually increases, ruling the body during the summer and autumn. The hot and dry summer weather is conducive to yellow bile, but as the cool and dry autumn comes on, the bile is cooled and the black bile preponderates, according to the popular reference *The Medical Works of Hippocrates: A New Translation from the Original Greek Made Especially for English Readers* (Oxford, England: Blackwell Scientific Publications, 1950), edited by John Chadwick, M.A., and W.N. Mann, M.D.

Because of these annual seasonal variations it is reasonable, noted Hippocrates, to expect most diseases to occur only during certain times of the year. Hence, in applying folk medical remedies, "The physician or common healer must bear in mind that each disease is most prominent during the season most in keeping with its nature." In addition, treatment should aim at opposing the cause of the disease: "Diseases caused by over-eating are cured by fasting; those caused by starvation are cured by feeding up. Diseases caused by exertion are cured by rest; those caused by indolence are cured by exertion. To put it briefly, the physician [*iatrós*] and common healer should [both] treat disease *by the principle of opposition* to the cause of the disease according to its form, its seasonal and age incidence, countering tenseness by relaxation and vice versa. This will bring the patient most relief and seems to me to be the principle of healing [itself]."

Since the important organs of the body (the heart, the brain, and the liver) were thought in classical Greek times to be respectively dry and hot, moist and cold, and hot and moist, the normal, healthy body had an excess of heat and moisture. But this balance varied with individuals, so that their temperaments, or [physical] "complexions," varied: the *sanguine,* ruddy, cheerful, optimistic; the *phlegmatic,* calm, composed, sluggish, apathetic; the *bilious,* choleric, ill-tempered; and the *melancholic,* depressed, sad, melancholic. Good medical practice in those distant times thus consisted of knowing the natural complexion of the patient to establish which humor or humors were momentarily excessive or deficient in quantity, matching these findings with the dominant humor of the season, and deciding how the normal humoral balance could best be reestablished. This was accomplished by means of diet, internal medicines, purging, vomiting, bleeding, cupping, and like forms of treatment.

The routes whereby classic Greek orthodox and folk medicines have come down to our times to produce contemporary folk humoral pathology are far too complex to mention here. Suffice it to say that Galen, the great Roman physician and recognized father of modern pathology, adopted many of these same Greek ideas into his own medical practice and gave them a final refinement, thereby assuring their supremacy for a long time to come. Through Byzantine civilization, Galen's influence was transmitted to the oriental Christians and to the Moslems. Some Muslim medical practitioners and folk healers carried these ideas westward into Spain and Italy.

Thus the ancient folk doctrine of humors became the basis of medieval Christian medicine, where it remained fairly dominant until the great medical discoveries of Vesalius (A.D. 1514–1564), who greatly advanced biology with his excellent descriptions and drawings of bones and the nervous system; Harvey (1578–1657), who made the wonderful discovery of how blood circulates; and Sydenham (1624–1689), who emphasized the importance of observation rather than theory in clinical medicine, which enabled him to make valuable epidemiological contributions in the treatment of gout, venereal disease, hysteria, fever, and epidemics. From the writings of Christian physicians and folk healers through this time, it is evident that Hippocrates, Galen, and certain Muslim practitioners were the principal authorities for medical theory and practice.

Even after its dethronement by scientific medicine, folk humoral pathology remained quite influential at the popular level until well into the nineteenth century in the form of herbals and home remedy books. From England, the American colonies also acquired the doctrine of humors. It continues to survive primarily among low-income blacks and poor white Southerners.

Little did the Greek doctors and folk healers realize in ancient times just how widespread their primitive humoral medical concepts would eventually become. It is in Latin America, however, that humoral medicine has had its greatest modern impact. With the discovery and conquest of the Americas, it came to the New World via the

Spanish *conquistadores* and later settlers. Parts of humoral pathology gradually filtered down from elitist medicine to the folk level, replacing, among Indian peasants, a large part of the pre-Conquest Aztec and Maya medicines and blending with those parts of both that managed to survive. Conforming to the processes whereby simplified parts of an elite culture eventually sift down to the level of the common people, humoral pathology lost the qualities of moist and dry.

Today in large parts of Latin America, from Mexico south through Hispanic and Portuguese South America, the folk variant of humoral pathology is the most important explanatory element in the medical systems of the rural—and to some extent the urban—peoples.

In contemporary Latin American humoral pathology, illness is ascribed to invasion of the body by excessive heat or cold. Sometimes actual temperature is involved, as when a woman explains hand and arm cramps as due to her carelessness in washing them in cold water when they were temporarily heated from ironing clothing. More often heat and cold are viewed metaphorically—a man who suffers hand and arm cramps may explain them as due to his carelessness in washing them when they were temporarily heated by the mineral lime he was using in whitewashing a wall. Cold may enter the body in the form of air, from the ingestion of "cold" foods, from stepping on a cold floor barefoot, and the like. Body heat rises from exposure to the sun, a potter's kiln, or a cooking fire, from bathing in warm water, from sleeping, from reading (the eyes become heated), from being pregnant or during the menses, from ingesting "hot" foods and beverages, and from experiencing "hot" emotions such as fright, anger, or grief.

In theory, illnesses believed to have hot causes are treated with cold herbal remedies, foods, and treatments (such as some kinds of skin plasters). Illnesses believed to come from cold causes are treated with hot herbal remedies, foods, and treatments (such as mustard plasters and cupping). In fact, most remedies are a mixture of a number of elements in which a hot or cold balance predominates.

The humoral pathology of the ancient Greek doctors and folk healers also diffused eastward, carried, as in the movement to the west, by the expanding Muslim empire. However, the version that accompanied this expansion was the one that had been shaped by Galen of Rome. From Iran, Pakistan, and other southwestern Asian nations, this version has demonstrated remarkable vitality at both sophisticated and folk levels. Today humoral pathology underlies much of the folk medicine in Malaysia, Indonesia, and the Philippines. In the Philippines these beliefs appear to be the result of Spanish influence. In contrast, Malaysian humoral pathology is clearly the result of Muslim influence. And the Javanese hot-cold syndrome of Indonesia, too, appears more nearly to correspond to the Muslim patterns than to indigenous south Asian influences. Thus, propelled eastward and westward by Muslim and Spanish influences, the basic Greek folk medical beliefs of classical times appear to have encircled the entire planet.

The Ayurvedic Medicine of Ancient India

In contemporary India, many foods are believed to have heating or cooling properties, and as in ancient Greek humoral pathology, the right combinations of foods and herbs can restore the proper balance when the body equilibrium has been disturbed. *Garam* (hot) foods include eggs, meat, milk, honey, and sugar; *tonda* (cold) foods include fruit juices, yogurt, buttermilk, rice, and water. These beliefs have their origin in Indian Ayurvedic medicine, an indigenous folk medical system that first appears in the Vedic literature of the early years of the first millennium B.C. These early texts, however, are as one scholar noted, "couched in terms of imprecations against demons, sorcerers, enemies; of charms for expelling diseases wrought by demons or sent by the gods as punishment for man's sin." It wasn't until significantly later that classical Ayurvedic medicine appeared in surviving Sanskrit documents: the *Caraka Samhita* of the first century A.D., the *Susruta Samhita* of about the fourth century A.D., and the *Vagbhata* of about the eighth century A.D. The theories found in these sources, however, certainly predate the sources by several centuries.

According to Ayurvedic folk medical theory, the universe is composed of the same four elements recognized by the Greeks—that is, earth, water, fire, and air—plus, a fifth one, ether. The arrangement in the body of these elements, each of which possesses five "subtle" and five "material" forms, reflects their arrangement in the universe. The human body also has three humors, or *dosha*: phlegm, or mucus; bile, or gall; and wind, or flatulence. Good health exists when the three dosha are in equilibrium; ill health manifests only when one or more of the dosha aren't functioning as they should. The dosha are also associated with age and the seasons: phlegm with youth and the growing season; bile with middle age and the rainy season; and wind with old age and cold, dry weather.

The similarities shared by Ayurvedic medicine and humoral pathology point to significant interrelationships between the two systems. Yet the historical record is such that mutual influences are difficult to prove until fairly late in time. Beginning early in the twentieth century, Ayurveda has become more and more important among Indian nationalists as a symbol of the antiquity and greatness of the Indian civilization. In fact, this is probably the only system of ancient folk medicine to have become a virtual lightning rod of national patriotism—from time to time the Indian National Congress has actively debated the logical merits of this folk healing system and elevated it to an almost official status by passing various laws to support and encourage it. This government championship of a particular folk medicine has sometimes been done almost to the supplanting of other forms of medical treatment.

There are some similarities between Greek humoral pathology and Indian Ayurvedic medicine. A court physician to a Persian emperor who was skilled in the Greek folk medical system made a visit to India sometime early in the sixth century A.D. While there he shared some of his medical knowledge with the physicians with whom he conferred and, in turn, received from the Indian physicians important information about the Ayurvedic methods of folk treatment. Thus, with this exchange of data, certain ideas from each folk medical system crept into the other over the course of time.

Whatever other historical relationships the two may have, Greek humoral pathology and Indian Ayurvedic medicine each have had their own distinct cultural histories. Whereas humoral pathology was developed and elaborated by a series of famous doctors in renowned medical centers, who then left us a massive written record, Hindu medical lore has been handed down through generations, not by faculties and bodies, colleges, or research centers, but through the individual training of pupils, considered to be masters of their craft. Yet today humoral pathology is folk medicine and an historical curiosity, while Ayurvedic folk medicine receives major Indian government funding as well as political backing. By the mid-1970s, there were 91 Ayurvedic medical colleges that were together admitting almost 7,000 students and had already trained about 50,000 "institutionally qualified" Ayurvedic physicians practicing a high form of distinguished folk medicine.

Traditional Chinese Medicine

The fourth and final great folk medical system of the ancient world to be examined here is traditional Chinese medicine (abbreviated here to TCM). TCM is best known through the *Huang Ti Nei Ching Su Wên,* the Yellow Emperor's "Inner Classic," or book of internal medicine. *Huang Ti,* the Yellow Emperor, was in Chinese genealogies the third of China's first five rulers; the precise dates of 2697–2597 B.C. are assigned to him. In fact, the book, while old, is considerably more recent. After sifting the evidence, scholars concluded that a great portion of the text existed during the Han dynasty (202 B.C.–A.D. 221), and that much of it is of considerably older origin, possibly handed down by oral tradition from China's earliest history. What this tells us is that ancient China's folk medical system began turning to naturalistic explanations at about the same time that the process also took place in Greece and India.

TCM represents a special case of the central concept of Chinese cosmology. This happens to be the dual forces of *yin* and *yang,* whose continuous interaction lies behind all natural phenomena, including the constitution and functioning of the human body. The proper balance within the body of yin and yang is essential for optimal health.

This principle of harmony, which views disease as essentially due to the disruption of harmony through internal or external, physical or mental causes, has remained central to all of later Chinese medicine.

Since yin and yang are believed to be the primordial elements from which the universe evolved, it isn't surprising that they are endowed with innumerable qualities. Their earliest meanings—cloudy and sunny—would today probably be interpreted by some psychotherapists and folk healers as "melancholy and cheery," to reflect the two main dispositions of mood that are considered the origins of poor and good health by many therapists. These early terms were eventually expanded over several millennia to produce a philosophical duality that can accommodate almost any concept.

Thus, yang signifies heaven, sun, fire, heat, dryness, light, the male principle, the exterior, the right side, life, high, nobility, good, beauty, virtue, order, joy, wealth—in short, everything positive. Yin represents just the opposite: earth, moon, water, cold, dampness, darkness, the female principle, the interior, the left side, death, low, ignobility, bad, ugliness, vice, confusion, and poverty—in other words, all of the negative things. Due to its heat, excessive yang causes fever; because of its coldness, excessive yin induces chills. Diseases believed to be caused by external forces are yang diseases, and those believed to be caused by internal forces are yin diseases. Yet yin and yang have always been conceived of as a single entity, combining, in any being or situation, both positive and negative elements.

Chinese philosophers (including TCM practitioners) recognized that five elements—water, fire, metal, wood, and earth—were all contained in the human body and were all linked to physiological processes and to specific internal organs. The number five was, in fact, the basis for an elaborate system of numerical concordances that described and integrated the entire universe, including man, so that most phenomena were thought to occur in sets of five. These phenomena included the seasons, directions, musical notes, colors, emotions, bodily orifices, food flavors, and internal organs. The linkage between the human body, health, and the universe is also found in the concordance of the number of days of the year with the 365 natural medicines of the earliest surviving pharmacopoeia and the 365 bodily surface points recognized for insertion of acupuncture needles.

The antiquity and importance of the hot-cold dichotomy in TCM has always been somewhat less than in the case of Greek humoral pathology and Indian Ayurvedic medicine. The hot-cold, wet-dry dichotomies, though, are implicit in the yin-yang duality. Yet in the Yellow Emperor's *Nei Ching* folk medicine treatise there are found no specific references to this particular belief. Instead, foods are classified according to five flavors (pungent, sour, sweet, bitter, and salty), and the proper manipulation of food involved balancing these flavors in much the same way that hot and cold foods were balanced in the previous two ancient folk medical systems.

Scattered bits of evidence extracted from a wide variety of Chinese medical literature appear to push a specific hot-cold dichotomy back as far as 180 B.C. For instance, heat and cold "condensed with moisture" in the intestines is a common explanation for intestinal worms. Far better evidence comes from Chia Ming's *Yin-shih-hsü* (*Essential Knowledge for Eating and Drinking*), dated at A.D. 1368. This remarkable treatise describes 43 kinds of fire and water, 50 types of grains, 87 kinds of vegetables, 63 types of fruits and nuts, 33 "flavorings" and condiments, 68 varieties of fish, 34 kinds of fowl, and 42 types of meat! The entry for each of these 460 items tells to which of the five flavor categories it belongs, its "character" (specified degrees of hotness or coldness), and the other foods that shouldn't be eaten with it. The character of natural rainwater, for example, is cold, while that of water from a stalactite cavern is warm; the flavor of both is sweet. Glutinous rice is said to be warm, and eaten in excess it causes fever. Soybeans and fragrant leeks are warm, vinegar is "slightly warm," and distilled spirits are "very hot." Spinach, persimmons, and milk are cold, on the other hand.

Whatever the time of the formalization of the hot-cold dichotomy in the Chinese dietary and medical systems, recent ethnographical work shows that the belief is widespread and pervasive today. Research that I've conducted in Hong Kong in the past as a medical anthropologist has demonstrated that a balance between heat and cold is considered essential to physical well-being. My investigations also have shown that foods and medicines have hot or cold qualities that must be taken into account when trying to maintain a proper balance in the diet and treat diseases. Moreover, acupuncture (the insertion of fine needles along the lines of the body's nerve "meridians") is a "cold" procedure, hence especially suited to those diseases attributed to a yang excess. Just the opposite of this, however, is moxibustion (the burning of tiny cones of dried leaves of mugwort on the skin), which is a "hot" treatment particularly suited to illnesses caused by too much yin.

In my travels throughout Hong Kong, China, Rangoon, Myanmar (formerly Burma), the city-state of Singapore, Jakarta, Indonesia, Bangkok, Thailand, Seoul, Korea, and Taipei, Taiwan, I've closely evaluated the diet and folk health beliefs and practices among many different Chinese-based communities. In such places hot foods are expanded to include strong alcoholic beverages, spicy and fatty foods, protein-rich dishes, and items prepared by long cooking at high heat (steaming, boiling, and baking). Cold foods include herbal teas, bland and low-calorie vegetables, beer, and the like. A few items, such as crabs, mollusks, and catfish, are both hot and wet; venereal diseases are "wet" and hot. The relative absence of good data on the hot-cold dichotomy in Chinese folk health beliefs is a consequence of past research neglect and not necessarily an absence of the trait itself.

Folk Medicine's "Great Tradition" Systems

The preceding text has briefly examined the folk medical systems of four of the world's ancient classic civilizations: Egypt, Greece, India, and China. By understanding something about each of them, it enables us to better appreciate the folk health beliefs in current existence among some of the world's different populations. Such a presentation has shown that some of these folk medical systems reach back a lot farther than most of us ever realized. We now have a better feel for the many modern variants that will be covered in the remaining chapters.

Chapter Two

THE MEDICINE OF
MY ANCESTORS

(Granny Remedies From Migratory Southern Whites)

The Other Grandmother

Every nuclear family in America has two sets of grandparents, those from the father's side and those from the mother's. In the Introduction I spoke somewhat about my father's mother, who emigrated with her husband and family from Hungary to the United States around 1904. She and the women seven generations before her possessed definite intuitive healing skills that could be favorably described as God-given in some ways. All of my father's people came from very traditional families and conservative European upbringing. These were people of values and definite roots, strong-willed individuals with a firm sense of commitment and deep attachment to community.

As my father, Jacob Heinerman, in his eighty-eighth year as of 2001, observed not too long ago: "Our people came from reliable stock, lived with purpose and meaning, and died in old age fully satisfied with everything they had accomplished." That heritage was reflected in the manner in which he was brought up and also the way he raised his two surviving sons (three children died in their infancy).

By contrast, my mother's people, all of whom were native-born Americans, came from less honorable backgrounds, but were also involved to some extent in natural healing circumstances. From old, brittle handwritten records that date back to about 1885 and were scribbled on cheaply made ruled paper by my "other grandmother," I am able to give something of their history here. Included with these documents is a time-worn, battered book containing a number of primitive medicinal remedies within its fragile pages.

Grandmother Elizabeth Jennie Webb Davidson, on my mother's side of the family, was born in July 1880 in Chestnut Hill, Tennessee, but spent most of her childhood and adulthood in the countryside within about a 100-mile radius of Houston, Texas. She passed away in 1950 in Salt Lake City, but was buried in Texas. Several of her close Tennessee relatives were what were called in those days in the Deep South "yarb and root" doctors, who specialized in the gathering of and doctoring with various botanicals indigenous to that part of the country. Grandma Elizabeth, as she preferred to be called, learned some of this at an early age before her parents again pulled up stakes for the umpteenth time and removed themselves to the Lonestar State in hopes of better fortunes. "We came to Texas in about 1885 or 1886," she penciled below some brief genealogical data concerning some of her kinfolk.

The historical narrative about herself and my mother, Jennie Faith Davidson Heinerman, which she managed to flesh out in the early months of 1933, reads like a drifter's guidebook of sorts, mentioning numerous towns that they settled in for short periods of time before moving on to somewhere else. While it may seem that my grandmother had a tad of gypsy blood in her to have been so mobile as she was, it was weather- and economic-related circumstances such as drought, flooding, grasshoppers, and dire poverty that accounted for much of this nomadic lifestyle.

Yet, it must be admitted that many of my mother's folks were—how shall I put it—rather strange people, to say the least. A stark illustration of this may be seen in the following little anecdote related to me by my father sometime ago. "Your mother's people were always a bit odd. When your Grandmother Elizabeth finally managed to come to Salt Lake City sometime in 1948 to visit her daughter, your mother and I drove down to the D&RG [Denver & Rio Grande] railroad depot to pick her up. Now, mind you, they hadn't seen or spoken to each other in almost five years. Your mother goes up to Elizabeth and demands in a businesslike tone of voice, 'Where's your bags and trunk?' There were no fond embraces or loving kisses, not even so much as a cordial 'hello' from either. That's just how they always were with each other."

Further proof of this is offered in something that my Grandmother Elizabeth wrote in her personal history. In an allusion to her own parents' compatibility, she mentioned that "Ma and Pa had relations only for the sake of getting children and nothing else!" Being brought up in an environment with little or no personal affection undoubtedly accounted for her own frequent infidelity in later married life; my own mother was born out of wedlock and never even knew who her real father was. She had numerous half-brothers and half-sisters fathered by different men other than the one to whom her own mother was legally married.

The Webbs and Davidsons were superstitious people who sometimes dabbled in the black arts. There is a passing reference made in Grandmother Elizabeth's papers to the effect that some of her relatives had occasionally resorted to metaphysical elements during the course of their folk medical doctoring. It was common for them to gather medicinal plants during periods of full moon and to compound some herbal formulas by magical chants. My own mother, Jennie Heinerman, during the course of her marriage to my father, Jacob, herself became involved with spiritualism to the point that she was taken over, or "possessed," by a malevolent entity of some kind, which finally resulted in her tragic suicide in January 1960 at the age of 39.

But on August 21, 1936, during her fifteenth year, she composed the little poem on page 28, which would have helped her greatly throughout her troubled life had she followed its inspired admonitions.

A DAILY PRAYER
by Jennie Davidson

Father hear this humble prayer,
As we bow before thy throne,
To whom we bring our care,
That thou wilt hear thine own.

We know that thou art true and kind,
And thou wilt hear our needs,
Father make clear our mind,
And answer not our lustful greeds.

Father, when we go astray,
Lead us back into thy way,
We know that thy almighty hand,
Will guide us to the promised land.

Granny Remedies from the Old South

Although my own mother never engaged in any kind of folk healing, nor ever had a mind to that I know of—her aptitude was more into science, linguistics, and history—her mother was somewhat of a practitioner of natural medicine.

The old, weather-beaten, and well-used remedy book kept by Grandmother Elizabeth and her mother was stored inside a manila envelope carefully tied with string to keep its contents together without being disturbed. Only when this writing project came along from my publisher did I retrieve it from its storage place and begin perusing its brittle pages.

Nothing really was in the order it should have been, probably typical of the lives of those folk healers, who kept and wrote in the book periodically. Their haphazard record keeping, however, wasn't without its benefits and advantages. Someone wrote an interesting treatise on a common aspect of folk medicine in general, which is reproduced here for the first time.

SOUTHERN DECOTIONS

The usual method of giving an herbal remedy is by means of what's known as a decoction. To make them, herbs are simply boiled by water. They should be prepared fresh daily. Sometimes herbs and water are boiled, strained and the liquor used to cover fresh herbs and again boiled. Decoctions should always be made over a clear flame or fire, free from wood smoke, in a covered vessel. In the case of herb leaves, brought to the boil, then strained into an earthenware jug and covered till cold.

Decoctions are solutions of the active principles of vegetable substances obtained by boiling. This method is adopted to obtain principles which can't be separated by simple infusion in cold or even boiling water. Small quantities only should be made at a time, as they are apt to change.

Decoction of oak bark—Take an ounce of oak bark and a pint of water. Put into a covered vessel and boil for 10 minutes, then strain. The dose of this preparation is from 2 to 6 tablespoonsful. It is a fine astringent and to be used as a gargle for relaxed throat.

Decoction of barley—Take 2 oz. pearl barley and 5 pints of water. Wash the barley in cold water, reject the washings, and having poured over it half a pint of water, boil for 5 minutes. Repeat, then after adding the remainder of the water boiling, let the whole boil down to 2 pints, then strain. Barley water made this way is serviceable in all cases of fever and inflammation, and can be taken in any quantity. To this, various substances are sometimes added, such as sliced figs, raisins, licorice root, slices of lemon, and sugar-candy.

Decoctions are valuable for illnesses connected with stomach, bowels and kidneys, because this fluid passes quicker into these organs than any other medicine. They can be sweetened with sugar but are better without. If roots, barks, leaves, flowers and seeds are boiled together, let the roots boil first for some time. Then add the bark and bring to the boil again. And so on with [the] leaves, seeds and flowers, each in the order given.

Figs, quince seeds, and linseed should be tied in a muslin

bag—all need long boiling—then should be removed before straining the liquid. Decoctions must be kept covered. The usual dose is
from 1 to 5 liquid ounces, according to the strength of the decoction
and the age of the patient.

Grandmother Elizabeth's Herbal Cupboard

The basis of my Grandmother Elizabeth's folk medicine capabili-
ties was—apart from a shrewd if untutored use of practical psychology—an encyclopedic knowledge of the curative value of herbs,
barks, and roots in general. What follows was written into the remedy
book handed down through several generations of Webbs and
Davidsons. Though some of them were certainly of her own creation,
many were contributed by some of our Tennessee relatives in the
early-to-mid-nineteenth century. I have carefully excerpted some of
the better ones that seem to be efficacious, simple to prepare, and safe
to use.

Rosemary decoction. A decoction of rosemary, made with wine
instead of water, is to be taken as a remedy against giddiness. A decoction of a good handful of the leaves, covered with cold water,
brought to the boil, and strained, is an excellent hair tonic to be
rubbed into the scalp till the skin nicely glows.

Balm. For stimulant to help fevers, try a compound spirit of
balm. This spirit—almost as good as a liqueur—is distilled from 8
ounces of balm, 4 ounces of lemon peel, 2 ounces each of nutmeg and
caraway seeds, and 1 ounce each of angelica root, cinnamon, and
cloves. Add a quart of brandy, keep the liqueur in stoppered bottles,
and use as a stimulant.

An infusion of balm is prepared by covering 1 ounce of leaves
with 1 pint of boiling water, and letting it stand for 15 minutes. Strain,
then take freely in wine-glassful doses as a tonic and to induce perspiration.

Beans. Beans good for a variety of problems. For boils, bruises, and blue marks caused by a blow; reduce haricot beans to a powder, mix with an equal quantity of fenugreek and honey, and apply to the affected area.

You can also treat eye troubles with beans. Mix bean flour with equal quantities of rose leaves and frankincense and the white of an egg. Apply to eyes that are tearing or swollen due to pollen allergies.

Sciatica can be eased by burning bean husks to ashes and mixing into an ointment with unsalted lard. Apply for old pains, sciatica, and gout.

Celery. This is excellent for rheumatism. Cut celery into pieces and boil in water until soft, then drink the water. Put fresh milk, with a little flour and nutmeg, into a saucepan with the boiled celery, and serve warm with pieces of toast. Eat with potatoes, and the rheumatic aches and pains will ease.

Chamomile lotion for hair and skin. Place 5 or 6 dried chamomile flowers into a bowl and pour a half pint of boiling water over them. Cover the bowl for 10 or 12 minutes. When the lotion has slightly cooled, sponge it on the skin with a small pad of cotton wool. Chamomile lotion is credited with astringent properties and is used for closing enlarged pores and toning up relaxed muscles. It also makes an excellent hair tonic. Cleanse the scalp with it twice a week.

Cherry juice. This is wonderful for curing gout, dropsy, and water retention. It also works well for rheumatism and arthritis. Remove the pits from four gallons of ripe cherries. Place the cherries into a muslin bag, tie the bag securely with string, and place the bag in a large square pan. With a rolling pin, roll back and forth over the top of the bag until all of the juice in the cherries has come out. Store the juice in an icebox. Bottled cherry juice works just as well.

Cold cream. To make a simple cold cream, take 1½ ounces of olive oil, 6 teaspoons of white candle wax, 2 teaspoons of spermacetti (a waxy solid obtained from sperm whale oil), and 3 drops of oil of lavender. Melt the wax and spermacetti in the oil in a double saucepan or a jar standing in a pan of boiling water over a flame. Stir vigorously with a porcelain or bone spoon (a wooden spoon will also do) until the ointment is well mixed. Remove the ointment from the fire and beat gently until it becomes stiff and sets, when it should be potted for use.

Coltsfoot. Coltsfoot syrup is a first-class remedy for coughs, colds, giddiness, and headache.

For coughs and colds make a decoction from a handful of the leaves in 2 pints of water. Boil down to 1 pint, strain, and sweeten with a syrup made of sugar-candy. The dose is an occasional teacupful.

Dandelion. Dandelion extract acts on the liver and has a slight purgative action on the bowels.

Boil down a decoction of the *fresh* root, sliced—1 ounce of root in 1 pint of water—to half a pint and strain. Then add 2 teaspoons of cream of tartar. Take a wine-glassful 2 or 3 times a day.

An excellent liver tonic is made from 4 ounces of fresh dandelion roots boiled in 2 pints of water until the liquid is reduced to 1 pint. Strain off and take a wine-glassful twice a day.

This is also good for rheumatism, stiffness in the joints, and sore muscles.

Ointment for obstinate ulcers. Lightly crush in a stone mortar with a pestle a pound of primrose leaves with half a pound of the flowers. Simmer them in an equal quantity of hog lard [Crisco shortening will do just fine] without salt until the primroses become crisp, then strain through a coarse sieve.

Elecampane. This root is aromatic, tonic, and stimulating. It is used for dyspepsia and pulmonary affections. It also works well for cases of hydrophobia resulting from the bite of a rabid dog or bat. Cousin Jesse Webb was cured of a case of this by drinking the infusion almost nonstop.

Infusion of elecampane is made from the dried root covered with boiling water; let sit for an hour or longer. Drink a wine-glassful every few hours for hydrophobia, including bites from diamond-back rattlers, common to the Texas prairies.

Hart's tongue.   A sure cure for hiccups. The distilled water of the hart's tongue fern is good for stopping even the worst case of hiccups that may result from sudden fright or a fearful lightning storm. Gradual sips is what's suggested. And used as a gargle, it's hard to beat for curing bleeding gums.

Lotion for soothing heat and skin irritation.   Take 2 ounces lettuce juice, 2 teaspoons of eau de cologne, 2 ounces distilled vinegar, and 4 ounces elder flower water, well mixed. Dab the skin with it frequently.

Lotion to soothe general body irritation.   Bathe with powdered boric acid diluted with an ounce of water, and powder afterward with talcum powder.

Linseed lotion.   For unbroken chilblains (itching and burning on the fingers, toes, heels, nose, and ears due to exposure to extreme cold) and rheumatism, apply a lotion made of 4 tablespoonsful each of pure linseed oil and oil of turpentine. Add 2 teaspoonsful of spirits of camphor and shake well until mixed.

Marshmallow ointment.   Highly prized for its soothing effects and for relieving inflammation. Make it by macerating equal weights of marshmallow leaves and pure unsalted hog lard [Crisco will do nicely here] together in a double saucepan or in a jar standing in a pan of boiling water. Simmer for an hour to extract all the soluble parts of the leaves before straining and potting the ointment.

Or boil the leaves for 45 minutes, strain and evaporate the liquid to a thin extract, and then mix with lard.

Kerosene.   Mix a couple of drops of coal oil or kerosene with a small pinch of sugar. Place on the end of the tongue and slowly suck. Be sure it mixes with plenty of saliva before swallowing each time. This will agitate the lungs just enough to cause them to cough up black or yellow mucus. Used in the coal mines of Tennessee and West Virginia to avoid getting black lung.

Remedies for Invalids

Those considered to be in an invalid condition may be temporarily disabled on account of sickness or extreme weakness but are not necessarily totally incapacitated. The following food items have been proven useful by Webb and Davidson folk healers in both Tennessee and Texas. They are safe, simple, and satisfying enough to guarantee rapid recuperation.

Arrowroot.   Take a tablespoon of arrowroot and mix it into a thin paste with a little water from the well bucket. Gradually add half a pint of boiling water, stirring the entire time. Put on the wood stove for several minutes, continuing to stir until the whole is evenly mixed.

Remove from the stove and add grated nutmeg, sugar, etc., to taste. A little lemon juice is a nice substitute for the nutmeg. The mixture is more nourishing if made with milk, but it can be too rich for a weak stomach, for which water is preferable. It should always be prepared fresh as required.

Although arrowroot is a valuable and easily digestible food for invalids and small children, remember that it isn't very nourishing. Flour tends to be more nutritive and less liable to ferment and is preferable over arrowroot.

Arrowroot pudding.   Rub a tablespoonful of arrowroot in a basin with a little cold water, and add, stirring constantly, a pint of boiling milk. Mix in the contents of an egg and 3 teaspoonsful of powdered, refined sugar, which have previously been beaten together. Boil in the basin or bake. This is good for early convalescence.

Arrowroot blancmange.   Take 3 tablespoonsful of arrowroot, make into a mucilage with water, then add milk in sufficient quantity and boil until of a proper consistency. Pour into a mold, and allow to cool and set. Eat with currant jelly or with lemon juice and sugar. Milk or beef tea may be used instead of water in the preparation of arrowroot mucilage. It should be boiled for 20 minutes. This again is excellent for early convalescence.

Arrowroot water.   Take 2 teaspoonsful of arrowroot, and make into a smooth paste with a little water. Add a pint of water, and simmer for 5 minutes, stirring constantly.

Strengthening jelly.   Soak overnight 2 ounces of isinglass (sturgeon gelatin) or regularly prepared gelatin, 1 ounce of gum arabic, 5 ounces of sugar-candy, and a grated nutmeg in a bottle of port wine. In the morning, simmer on the wood stove till dissolved. Strain and set aside in a cool place till it forms into firm jelly. A piece the size of a nutmeg may be taken 5 or 6 times a day. This is good for debility when the stomach is unable to bear normal food.

Strawberry tea.   Strawberries contain citric acid, and "strawberry treatment" is something the Webbs and Davidsons have found very effective for gout, stone in the bladder, kidney trouble, stone in the kidneys, and worms in the intestines.

In fever cases, strawberries squeezed in water make a cooling, refreshing beverage. A delightful-tasting tea can be made from the dried leaves of wild strawberries. May and June are the best months to collect the leaves. At the same time, collect young blackberry leaves and young wood-roof leaves [specific identity unknown], and dry in the same way as the strawberry leaves. From a mixture of these three kinds of leaves, you can produce a drink equal in taste and aroma to Chinese tea.

Young blackberry leaves possess the same taste as pure, good Chinese tea leaves, and make a tea that is better than most other teas. The leaves must be put in a dry place, not in the sun, then stored for use in a closed jar. To make about 6 cups of tea, use as much as can be taken up with the tips of the fingers of one hand. Pour boiling water on it, and leave for 5 or 10 minutes. Add a little sugar, but no milk, and you have a very pleasant-tasting drink.

Hive honey. Honey is an excellent "pick-me-up" for older folks. It is laxative, purifying, and strengthening. Mixed with tea, it is a remedy for catarrh (simple inflammation of a mucous membrane) and phlegm. It is also good for external sores if you take half-parts of honey and flour and mix them well together with a little water. Honey ointment should be thick, not fluid. Used internally, honey acts effectively in many other ailments, too.

If difficulty of swallowing is felt, boil a teaspoonful of honey with half a pint of water. This makes a delicious throat gargle for singers; and if a drop is swallowed, there is no risk of tummy upset.

Honey water is wonderful for the eyes as a purifier and strengthener. Boil a teaspoonful of honey in half a pint of water for 5 minutes, and the decoction is ready for use.

My grandmother Elizabeth Webb Davidson knew a man of 90 years of age who added a teaspoonful of pure honey to some boiling water and allowed it to boil for a time. He soon had a tasty wine that was also invigorating. He used to tell her, "I owe my strength and vigorous old age to this honey-wine." Its effects are mildly purgative to the bowels, purifying to the blood, nourishing to the system, and invigorating overall. It is reminiscent of the "mead" of ancient days.

Honey is excellent for healing an ulcerated throat. Boil a spoonful of honey in 2 pints of water for a few minutes, then take 2 to 4 spoonsful of it every hour.

A good stomach remedy is half a spoonful of coriander boiled with a spoonful of honey in 2 pints of water. A spoonful taken hourly cleanses the stomach.

Weak, delicate children should be given a cupful or two of boiled milk daily to which has been added a little honey. Never use raw honey for a cough as it can sometimes be a tad too sharp, but if boiled in either well water or cow's milk, it will sooth or clear up the cough completely.

Brandy mixture.   Beat 2 egg yolks and a half-ounce of powdered white sugar together. Add 4 tablespoons of brandy and water, flavor with grated cinnamon and nutmeg, and you have a wonderful stimulant and restorative for anyone feeling run down.

The adult dose should be from 1 to 3 tablespoonsful repeated according to need. Children should be given a teaspoonful to a tablespoonful according to age.

White wine whey.   Take a pint of milk and add mace, nutmeg, and cinnamon with sugar to taste. Heat until the milk is on the verge of boiling. Remove from the heat and add in 1 or 2 wine-glassfuls of sherry or white wine. Put back on the boil, stirring gently one way until it curdles. Remove, and strain through a teacloth or some muslin. Make sure the patient is warmly tucked into bed, then give him this mixture and it will make him perspire freely. This is wonderful for catarrh and influenza.

Wine whey.   Pour half a pint of sherry into a pint of boiling milk. Stir thoroughly until it coagulates. Strain off the whey, and sweeten to taste.

Egg nog.   Beat an egg yolk with 6 ounces of milk. Add some brandy or whiskey, and some sugar. Add a beaten egg white. A tablespoonful of lime juice added to wine whey and egg nog makes them both more easily digested.

Egg jelly.   Take 3 newly laid eggs from the hen house. Separate the whites from their yolks, and beat separately. Dissolve half an ounce of isinglass or prepared gelatin in a quarter pint of warm water and add the juice of half a lemon. Mix together and add 2 tablespoonsful of brandy. Pour into a mold and cool in the ice box.

Pish-pash.   For invalids, pish-pash is fresh meat cooked in rice. Cut a chicken into small pieces, place in a small pan, and add 3 tablespoonsful of rice. Pour over it 2 coffee cupsful of cold water, and cook slowly. You can add spices during cooking. The rice, which will have absorbed most of the strength of the meat, can be used alone if the patient is very ill.

Water-souchy.   Take 2 flounders, soles, or haddocks, and boil them in a quart of water until they are reduced to mere pulp; strain. Remove the fins from 4 more fish and put the additional fish into the liquid. Add pinches of salt and cayenne pepper to taste and a little chopped parsley. Boil well and eat with the sauce. This is very digestible and helps invalids in their recuperation from long-term sickness and/or recent surgery of some kind.

Macaroni pudding.   To 4 tablespoonsful of cinnamon water add 2 ounces of macaroni. Simmer until the macaroni is tender. Add 3 egg yolks, the white of an egg, an ounce of sugar, a drop of oil of bitter almonds, and a glass of raisin wine beaten into half a pint of milk. Bake in a slow oven.

Rice pudding.   Add 2 tablespoonsful of rice to a pint and a half of milk and simmer until the rice is soft. Add 2 eggs beaten with half an ounce of sugar. Bake for three-quarters of an hour in the oven.

Rice and apples.   Take some rice and boil quickly in hot water. Strain through a colander; expose for 15 minutes. Stew separately some apples, then mix with the rice and sweeten to taste.

Rennet whey.   Take a piece of rennet and infuse it in some boiling water, removing all the soluble matter. After pouring off the liquid, take a tablespoonful of it and mix this with 3 tablespoonsful of milk. Place the mixture near heat, covering it with a piece of clean cloth. When a uniform curd forms, remove it from the heat, divide it into small pieces with a spoon, and separate the whey with gentle pressure. This is good for feverish conditions.

White wine whey.   Put a half pint of fresh milk into a deep pan. Place on the stove, and as soon as the scrum rises to the edge of the pan, pour in a glass of sherry or other white wine, and sweeten with a teaspoonful of refined sugar. Boil again, stirring constantly, then place aside until the curd forms a lump. Strain the whey through a sieve or piece of muslin. It can be taken cold or tepid and is an excellent moderate stimulant.

Egg brandy.   Take 3 eggs and beat them with 5 ounces of plain water. Slowly add 3 ounces of brandy, as well as a little sugar and nutmeg. Take two tablespoonsful of this at a time. It is good for prostration cases in which the invalid is doubled over due to severe abdominal or other pain.

Another useful stimulant is made by taking the white of a new-laid hen's egg and stirring it with a tablespoonful of cream. Add a tablespoonful of brandy in which a lump of sugar has been dissolved.

Milk and soda water.   Sweeten half a pint of milk with a teaspoonful of refined sugar. Bring almost to the boiling point and pour a bottle of soda water over it. For stomach acidity, this is the way to administer milk.

Boiled flour and milk.   Knead wheaten flour with water, put it into a linen cloth, and tie firmly. Place it in a pan of water and boil it slowly for 12 hours. Dry, then take the thick rind away on removing the cloth, and again dry. A tablespoonful of this grated and boiled with a pint of milk is excellent for recovery from diarrhea or dysentery.

Boiled bread pudding.   Pour a pint of hot milk over half a pound of stale bread and allow the mixture to soak for an hour in a covered basin. Beat with 2 eggs. Put it all into a covered basin, tie a cloth over it, and place it in boiling water for half an hour. Eat with salt or sugar.

Batter pudding.   Beat the contents of 2 eggs with half an ounce of sugar. Mix this with a tablespoonful of wheaten flour and a pint of milk. Put in a basin of boiling water and boil with a cloth tied over it.

Tapioca pudding.   Make a pint of tapioca mucilage with milk.

Beat 2 egg yolks with half an ounce of sugar, and stir into the mucilage. Bake in a slow oven. Sago and arrowroot can be made into similar puddings.

Mashed carrots and turnips.   Peel the carrots and turnips, boil separately in 3 successive waters, press the water out through a clear, coarse cloth, and mash together with sufficient milk to make into a pulp. Season with salt. Place in an enamel pan in a moderately heated oven till the surface dries over.

Vermicelli or macaroni soup.   Make some beef tea by boiling a few soup bones, an ox tail, or a beef tongue in one and a half quarts of water for 45 minutes, until the amount is reduced down to just a quart. Strain off one-third of the liquid and store the rest in the icebox, toward the back, if possible, where it's usually the coldest. (Make sure the ice man has brought you a fresh block of ice to put in the top of your icebox so that it will keep things stored below much cooler than if there was less ice.)

Bring the one-third quart of beef tea to another boil and add an ounce of vermicelli or 2 ounces of macaroni previously well boiled in other water. Boil the whole down to 1 pint. Add salt to taste. Instead of vermicelli or macaroni, you can use rice, but add the rice after the soup has been concentrated. Prepare the rice by boiling and slightly drying it.

Chicken broth.   Beat the yolk of an egg with 2 ounces of water. Add along with parsley or celery to chicken tea, and boil to half. Rice, vermicelli, or macaroni, fully boiled, can be mixed in.

Mutton broth with vegetables.   Slowly boil in a pan for 2 hours a pound of fat-free mutton chops. Remove the chops, and to the remainder add 3 carrots and 3 turnips, peeled, sliced, boiled, with the water drained, plus 2 onions, sliced and boiled. Season with salt and celery. Simmer slowly for 4 hours. Put the chops in again and simmer for another hour.

Tripe.   Boil some onions in 2 quarts of water and partially boil some tripe. Boil together slowly until the tripe is soft and tender. Add salt and a small pinch of cayenne pepper. Tripe is easily digested and very good for anyone convalescing from a bout of sickness or physical weakness and in need of regaining strength.

Grit-gruel.   This is an old family remedy that came from Georgia during the Civil War to the Webbs in Tennessee and traveled with them to Texas, where it became a part of the Davidson folk healing practices.

Wash grits in cold water. Pour off the fluid and add fresh cold water. Boil slowly until the water is reduced by half, then strain through a sieve. An ounce and a half of grits should make a pint of gruel.

Oatmeal gruel.   Take 2 or 3 tablespoonsful of oatmeal and rub in an enamel pan with a little cold water. Repeat the process, adding fresh water each time until the milkiness stops reaching the water. Put these washings into another pan and boil them on the range till a thick mucilage forms. These gruels contain more nourishment than sago, arrowroot, or tapioca, as they contain a small quantity of gluten. Sweeten the gruel and mix it with milk, if preferred.

Iceland jelly moss.   Iceland moss contains a bitter principle that should be cleared before use. To do this, pound the moss dry; soak it in tepid water with a little bicarbonate of soda for 24 hours, then press it through a coarse cloth. Add an ounce of the prepared moss to a quart of water and let the mixture boil to a half. Strain through a sieve and sweeten or mix with milk, according to the individual taste of the patient you're treating.

(Author's note: Iceland moss is a common remedy in the British Isles and Scandinavia, where it has been an effective treatment for constipation, dysentery, tuberculosis, and bronchitis.)

Folk Tonics for Convalescents

As with the foregoing "Remedies for Invalids," the Webb-Davidson folk healers on my mother's side of the family developed, over the course of several generations, a number of food-and-beverage tonics that were frequently employed with those in debilitated conditions or frail states of poor health, or otherwise suffering from general exhaustion.

As I've carefully gone through the remedy book that my grandmother Elizabeth Webb Davidson and her people kept, it has become abundantly clear that the greater majority of their treatments were for those confined to bed, disabled in some way, experiencing unsound health, under a doctor's or nurse's care, or even, in some instances, paralyzed. The tonics presented here for the very first time are "tried-and-true" in every sense of the word and brought about varying degrees of recuperation for the physically enfeebled and nutritionally devitalized.

They can be used with a full guarantee as to their safety and an absolute guarantee of expectation in their efficacy, too.

Cranberry drink.   Mash a teacupful of cranberries into a cup of water. Boil 2 quarts of water with a large spoonful of oatmeal and a bit of lemon peel. Add the cranberries and some sugar, then about one-quarter pint or less of sherry. Boil the whole for half an hour and strain off.

Egg milks.   Beat a fresh-laid hen's egg and mix it well with one-quarter pint of warm milk, a tablespoonful of rose petal water, and a little scraped nutmeg. Do not warm the mixture after the egg is mixed in. Taken first thing in the morning and last thing at night, it will be found strengthening and particularly helpful for anyone suffering from a cough. [Author's note: Raw eggs may be contaminated with Salmonella, a bacteria that causes food poisoning.]

Add the beaten yolks of 3 eggs to 2 tablespoonsful of powdered white sugar, 3 cloves, the rind of half a lemon, and half a pint of brandy. Pour a quart of warm milk over it, stirring rapidly. Serve immediately.

Strengthening drink for incapacitated patients.   Beat an egg white to a froth, then beat the yolk in a tablespoonful of cold water. Put another tablespoonful of cold water in a wineglass, add a tablespoonful of sherry, and make hot. Pour in the egg yolk, put in a saucepan, and stir constantly over a slow flame. Stir one way till it thickens; do not let it boil. When hot, put in the whipped white to set. The drink can be taken hot or cold.

Parsley tea.   This stimulates the kidneys and is good for rheumatism. Take a handful of freshly gathered leaves or a tablespoonful of dried parsley, and wash in cold running water. Put into an earthenware jug and pour over a pint of boiling water. Cover the jug with a cloth. Let the mixture get cold, then strain it into a glass jug. Drink plenty of it an hour before meals.

Peppermint tea.   Infuse a large handful of mint leaves in half a pint of boiling water, then add a teaspoonful of honey. A wineglassful taken hot at bedtime is excellent for a cold.

For cases of nausea and flatulence, add an ounce of mint leaves to a pint of boiling water. Let stand till cold, strain, and take a wineglassful frequently.

Hawthorn tea.   Mix hawthorn leaves together with balm and sage, about a half handful of each. Add to 1 quart of boiling water, cover, and set aside to steep for half an hour. This tea soothes the nerves of people who have been sick for a long time.

Ground rice milk.   Mix a tablespoonful of ground rice with a pint and a half of mokk, add half an ounce of lemon peel dipped in sugar water and cut into slices, then boil for half an hour; strain while still hot. This is nutritious during acute disease stages and early convalescence.

Rice milk.   Boil a tablespoonful of ground rice with a pint and a half of milk or equal parts of milk and water. Stir smooth and boil for 2 minutes. Flavor with sugar and nutmeg. This is very nourishing for sick children.

Bread panada.   Grate a piece of stale bread and mix it into sufficient water to form a thick pulp. Cover, and after it has soaked for an hour, beat it with 2 tablespoonsful of milk and a little sugar, then boil it for 10 minutes, stirring constantly.

Sago drink.   Add a tablespoonful of the best sago to a pint of water and let it stand for two hours, then boil it for a quarter of an hour, stirring constantly until it forms a clear, uniform jelly.

Remove from the stove and flavor with sugar and nutmeg, as in the case of arrowroot (see page 34). Instead of water you can use milk. Sago is frequently employed when a nonstimulating diet is required.

Sago milk.   Soak an ounce of sago in a pint of water for an hour. Pour off the water and add a pint and a half of milk. Boil slowly until the sago is well incorporated into the milk.

Sago posset.   Put 2 tablespoonsful of sago into a pint of water and boil until a mucilage forms. Take lemon rind and rub a quarter ounce of loaf sugar on it. Add 5 ounces of sherry wine along with half a teaspoonful of tincture of ginger. Add the mixture to the sago mucilage and boil for 5 minutes. A wine-glassful may be taken at a time and is excellent for debility from acute diseases of a noninflammatory nature.

(*Author's note*: The sago referred to in the foregoing remedies was quite common in the latter part of the nineteenth century and first four decades of the twentieth century as both a food and a medicinal agent. Sago is a dry granulated or powdered starch prepared from the pith of a sago palm.)

Tapioca.   Prepare the same as sago. However, since it is more soluble in water, macerate and boil for only half the time. Sweeten and flavor as you would sago.

Motherwort tea.   Place a full tablespoonful of dried motherwort herb in a ceramic or stone jug, and then pour a cupful of boiling water over it. Cover the jug with a cloth and leave to cool. Strain, then divide into two doses and take at half-hour intervals. This is a good stimulant for tired mental workers or those suffering from "brain exhaustion."

Sage tea.   Boil equal parts of sage, rosemary, honeysuckle vine, and plantain in water. Be sure the water covers the contents thoroughly. Add a tablespoonful of honey to each pint of liquid you get and use as required. This makes a wonderful gargle for sore throats, a soothing tonic for distressed lungs, and a gentle healer for a sore mouth, not to mention a great hairwash.

Yarrow tea.   Brew as you would ordinary tea, with a tablespoonful each of dried yarrow leaves and elder flowers placed in a pint of boiling water, covered, and set aside to steep for 20 minutes. Drink hot on retiring if you have a bad head cold.

Lime water.   Excellent to give to children with their milk when there is a tendency to acidity or when the bowels are too relaxed. Mix a tablespoonful of freshly squeezed lime juice with 3 tablespoonsful of milk.

Apple water.   Slice 2 large apples and pour a quart of boiling water on them. Let sit for 2 or 3 hours, strain, and sweeten with honey.

Linseed tea.   Take 2 teaspoons of bruised licorice root and an ounce of linseed, and put into a pint of boiling water. Allow to stand near a warm stove for 4 hours, then strain through muslin or calico. Don't bruise the linseed, though. This tea is good for coughs, sore throat, inflamed lungs, and hoarseness.

Egg wine.   Beat an egg (yolk and white together) with a tablespoonful of cold water. Pour on it a heated mixture of a glass of sherry or white wine and half a glass of water, stirring all the time. Sweeten with white sugar and add a little grated nutmeg to taste. Taken in this form, egg wine is more digestible. However, the flavor can be improved by heating it in a saucepan (not to the boiling point, however), stirring it one way for a minute till thickened. With a slice of toast or biscuit, this can be advantageously taken by invalids twice daily. [Author's note: Raw eggs may be contaminated with Salmonella, a bacteria that causes food poisoning.]

Lemon whey.   Pour as much lemon juice into boiling milk as will make a small quantity quite clear. Dilute with hot water to an agreeable acid, and put in a pinch of sugar. This promotes perspiration.

Egg emulsion.   Rub the yolks of 2 eggs and a little sugar with a pint of cold water using the back of a wooden spoon. Afterward, add a glass of wine and a little lemon juice for flavor. This is very restorative in cases of debility and for recovery from severe illness when mild stimulation is required. With wine, the emulsion is good for coughs, hoarseness, and constipation.

Toast and water.   Toast very brown 1 pint of white or brown breadcrusts in the top of a wood range oven on a flat metal sheet. Add a pint of cold water, and let stand an hour. Strain, then add cream and sugar.

Apple tea.   Roast 2 large sour apples and cover with boiling water. Cool, strain, and add sugar to taste.

Rice water.   Put 2 tablespoonsful of rice in 1 quart of cold water; cook an hour or until dissolved. Add salt and sugar to taste.

Flaxseed lemonade.   Pour a quart of boiling water over 4 tablespoonsful of cold flaxseed. Steep for 3 hours, strain, add the juice of 3 freshly squeezed lemons, and sweeten to taste.

Orange whey.   Add the juice of a freshly squeezed orange to a pint of sweetened milk. Heat slowly until curds form. Strain and cool.

Egg lemonade.   Take the white of an egg, 1 tablespoonful of powdered sugar, the juice of 1 lemon, and 1 glass of water, and beat together with a fork.

Baked milk.   Put half a gallon of milk in a jar and tie it down with some heavy butcher paper, several brown-paper shopping bags, or several layers of old newsprint. Let it stand in a moderate oven for 8 to 10 hours. It will be like cream and very nutritious.

Cranberry jelly juice.   Mix cranberry jelly with cold water.

Red currant whisky.   For a cold, add a little red currant jelly to a glass of hot whiskey punch. Drink before going to sleep.

Homemade lemonade.   Hot, strong lemonade at bedtime will often break up a bad cold. Add the juice of 3 freshly squeezed lemons to a pint of hot water, flavor with a pinch of sugar or one-quarter teaspoon of honey, and drink before retiring.

Imperial drink.   To a quart of boiling water add 2 teaspoonsful of cream of tartar and the juice of 2 freshly squeezed lemons, and sweeten with honey or sugar to taste. Allow to cool before drinking.

Barley water.   Add 1 tablespoonful of pearly barley to a pint of water and boil for a few minutes, stirring constantly to wash the grain. Pour off the water and add a pint and a half of clean water. Simmer gently for an hour and strain. Add sugar and lemon juice to taste, if desired. This is extremely good for colds and other illnesses.

Steak tea.   Take a pound of beefsteak and mince or cut it into small pieces; put it in a well-covered jar with a pint and a half of cold water or barley water. Now place the jar in a saucepan of water and simmer for 3 hours, or leave the jar in a not-too-hot oven overnight. Strain, and remove any fat.

Or take some good-quality beefsteak; beat it well, rub pepper and salt over it, place it on a flat tin punched with small holes (an onion grater can be used), pour some port wine over the meat, then cover it with a plate and place some weights on it. Increase the weights a couple of times to help press all the juice from the meat.

Chicken tea.   Take a small chicken. Remove the skin and the fat from between the muscles, and divide the chicken into two long halves. Remove the lungs and everything adhering to the backbone and chest walls; cut the meat into thin slices. Place the slices in a pan with some salt, then pour a quart of boiling water over them. Cover the pan and boil slowly for 2 hours. Allow to stand for half an hour, then strain off the fluid through a sieve. Steak tea and chicken tea are excellent during sickness if an animal diet is permitted and, by adding flour or another thickening substance, are good convalescence nourishment.

Mutton tea.   Cut a pound of mutton, free of fat, into thin slices. Pour a pint and a half of water over it, allowing it to macerate, as when making steak tea. Afterward, boil the mixture for half an hour and then strain.

Veal tea.   Slice a pound of filet of veal, free of fat, then boil it for half an hour in a pint and a half of water.

Stokos.   Put three-quarters pound of fine oatmeal, 6 ounces sugar, and half a lemon cut into slices into a pan. Mix together with a little warm water. Add a gallon of boiling water, stir thoroughly, and drink cold. This is a very nourishing beverage, as is the next suggestion.

Cokos.   Mix into a thin batter 6 ounces of sugar, 6 ounces of fine oatmeal, and 4 ounces of cocoa. Add a gallon of boiling water, put into a stone or earthenware bottle, and cork. This is a very good drink after doing strenuous work.

Mustard bath. Finally, for the convalescent, there is the mustard bath, which is also a wonderful stimulant to soak in but not to be taken internally as a fluid beverage. Two tablespoonsful of mustard are needed for every gallon of water to be used in the bath. The mustard should first be made into a paste in a pan, then gradually added to the water in the bath. The suggested water temperature is about 100°F.

Proper Breathing, Indian Style

My mother's grandmother, Sarah Elizabeth Kelly Webb, was born in Chestnut Hill, Tennessee, on July 26, 1863, and died March 4, 1918, in Brownwood, in central Texas. She knew or somehow made contact with George Catlin, an American artist and author, about a year before his death, in the company of her Grandmother Kelly (by whom she had been adopted in infancy).

At the time of their meeting she was still fairly young, about 7 or 8 years of age. But she distinctly remembered some of the things that this elderly gentleman told her grandmother and her about his many years' association with a variety of American Indian tribes, many of whom he drew sketches and portraits illustrating their unique way of life and customs.

One of the things that clearly stuck in her young mind for the rest of her life was his emphasis on correct breathing; Catlin, she wrote in her brief life history later on, had concluded that one of the chief causes of ailments affecting civilized peoples is their habit of breathing through the mouth.

The Indian child, he claimed, as she wrote from memory, was never allowed to sleep with his or her mouth open. The mother would always press the baby's lips together as soon as it fell asleep, to form a lasting habit of learning to breathe through its nostrils instead. So, when the child grew to adulthood, whether sleeping or waking, he or she kept the mouth closed at all times. Mr. Catlin claimed that this habit was the reason why the native races of North and South America used to enjoy such good physical perfection and escaped so many of the diseases of civilized communities. Among several million native Indians throughout the Americas, he never saw or heard of a hunchback or crooked spine, or an idiot or lunatic, and premature death was also quite uncommon.

My great-grandmother Sarah Webb wrote these words in her short bio, but whether they are Catlin's or her own cannot be identified with certainty. Nevertheless, I give them here just as she placed them in her personal history:

It is plain that nostrils are meant for breathing, and are the natural outlet of the lungs. The sides of the air passages are lined with hair which, to some degree, prevent ingress of noxious matters. You are healthier if you breathe through the nose. Some people who lived in malarious districts for years without suffering from any of the fevers that haunt such neighborhoods, ascribe their exemptions entirely to the habit of breathing properly. Air comes in contact with the membranes of the nose, and they are supposed to have some power of neutralizing malarious and contagious poisons. It is also to be noticed that, by drawing in our breath only through the nostrils, the air is warmed by contact with the membranes before it reaches the lungs, and so inflammation and congestion of these organs are avoided.

Perfect sleep cannot be obtained with the mouth wide open. Contrast the natural repose of the Indian child, which has been educated to keep its lips closed, with the uncomfortable slumbers of the child of civilization, with its little mouth wide open and gasping for breath. The firmly shut mouth, too, promotes good looks. Who ever yet saw an open mouth that was not insipid and unattractive? Keep your mouth shut, then, when you read, when you write, when you listen, when you are in pain, when you are walking, when you are running, and by all means when you are angry.

All crooked or constrained bodily positions affect aspiration. Reading, writing, sitting, standing, speaking, or working with the trunk of the body bent forward is extremely hurtful, by overstretching the muscles of the back, compressing the lungs, and pushing downward and backward the stomach, bowels, and abdominal muscles.

By following these few simple instructions that she had learned from Mr. Catlin, my great-grandmother Sarah Webb wrote that almost anyone could have good health. She and my grandmother Elizabeth Jennie Webb Davidson practiced a kind of benevolent folk medicine for which they charged little or nothing at all. And while their people were considerably migratory by habit and couldn't stay planted for very long, they contributed much to the relief of the suffering humanity with whom they came in contact. Their many small and sometimes great acts of kindness were obviously remembered by those they treated, which undoubtedly has earned for them lovely rewards in the life hereafter.

Chapter Three

THE ETHNOBOTANY OF BLACK AMERICANS

PART I: FOLK MEDICINE OF THE EARLY SLAVES

(Barbados, Dominican Republic, Haiti, Jamaica, and the Lesser Antilles)

Discovery of the Americas

It is a well-established fact that there were men of all sizes, features, and complexions in the Americas before 1492. Several tribes—the Choco, the Manabis, and the Yarura, to mention just a few—were as black as the African slaves that followed a few short years later.

Under the heading of fortuitous visits to the American continent prior to that of Columbus, Pietro Martire d'Angheira (Peter Martyr, 1457–1526), the earliest historian of the Americas, mentions an event that took place at Quarnea, in the Gulf of Darien, where Vasco Nuñez de Balboa met with a colony of Africans. By what means they had come to that region and how long they had resided there are not recorded by the Spanish historian. But it was surmised that because of the smallness of their number they must have arrived upon the coast relatively recently. There can be no doubt that their journey from Africa was accidental, for they were in open canoes of no stronger construction than those of the American Indians.

The modern history of the New World begins with Columbus, who sailed from Palos, Spain, with two caravels and a decked ship, on August 3, 1492, under the patronage of King Ferdinand and Queen

Isabella of Castile and Aragon. On October 12, in the same year, he landed on one of the islands of the Bahamas, which he called San Salvador. With that unique event, the European discovery and exploration of the New World began.

Cuba was the next island of importance to be discovered. This was followed by the discovery of Santo Domingo, now divided into the Dominican Republic and Haiti, where the Spanish formed a colony among the island's inhabitants and renamed the island Española or Hispañiola. In the three succeeding voyages of Columbus, the mainland of South America near Trinidad as well as several other islands were explored. These explorations eventually culminated in the colonization of Cuba, Jamaica, Trinidad, Puerto Rico, and finally Mexico and Peru.

The Commencement of Slavery in the New World

Hispaniola, or to be exact Santo Domingo, was the first land colonized by the Europeans in the New World. This was the starting point of the new civilization, which spread quickly throughout the Western hemisphere. It was there that enslaved Africans were introduced into the Americas, and there, too, strangely enough, that emancipation was first proclaimed.

As early as 1502, the Spanish began to use Negroes in the mines of Hispañiola. A year later Nicolás de Ovando, the governor of the island, forbade further importations of Africans, alleging that they taught the native Indians, also slaves, all manners of wickedness and rendered them less tractable. The decrease of the Indians for varied reasons induced the court of Spain, a few years later, to revoke the orders issued by Ovando, and to authorize, by royal decree, the introduction of African slaves from the Portuguese settlements on the coast of Guinea (West Africa). In 1517 Charles V of Spain ordered that 4,000 Negroes were to be supplied annually to the islands of Hispaniola, Cuba, Jamaica, and Puerto Rico. With that decree the supplying of Negroes to the Spanish-American plantations became an established and regular branch of commerce.

The unaccustomed labor of planting and cutting sugarcane, digging in the mines, and other drudgeries had quickly undermined the resistance of the native Indian slaves, who were also cruelly treated. Their bodies were neither of the athletic type, nor were they capable of enduring the fatigue of hard labor, so that their spirits were quickly broken in consequence. It was for this reason that the Spanish colonists had gone to the Portuguese coast of Africa for Negro laborers. The climate of Hispaniola proved so benign and natural to the blacks that it was commonly said "that unless one of them happened to be hanged for a particular crime, none ever died there."

Sugar and the traffic in Negro slaves were introduced to Jamaica as soon as the colony was able to assume the responsibilities involved. Here and elsewhere the Negro slave became an increasingly important factor as, by degrees, the native Indians became almost extinct on all of the larger islands, partly by their escaping to the continent, and partly as a result of their cruel treatment at the hands of their new lords.

The inhabitants of Jamaica were varied. Europeans, as well as Creoles, who were born and bred in Barbados, in the Windward Islands, or in Surinam, were the masters; the Indians, Negroes, mulattoes, Alcatrazes, mestizos (Euro-Indians), and cuarterones (three-quarters white and one-quarter black), to mention a few, were always the slaves.

The Negroes were of several types: Those from the different parts of Guinea (West Africa) were considered the best slaves, while those from the East Indies or Madagascar were considered merely adequate. Because the latter were accustomed to eating fresh meat in their own countries, they often died as a result of the lack of this important dietary element. Those who were born on the island or taken from the Spanish were thought to be worth more than all the others, for they were acclimatized to life on the islands.

A Typical Life in Slavery

The change from Africa to Santo Domingo was but very slight. The plantation slaves retained all the traits of their native cultures, including the religious basis of voodoo, their original language and dress, and as some allege, even cannibalism in a few instances. The damp forests supplied them with a natural environment very similar to that from which they came, and they continued to live in African-style huts and to eat African-style foods. The French masters practiced, under the guise of civilization, all the cruelties of some African rulers. The French system of slavery was unsurpassed for severity, subtle cruelty, lasciviousness, and ferocity. A marked contrast could be seen on the other (eastern) side of the island, in Santo Domingo, where the Spanish form of Negro slavery was, by comparison, much less severe.

In 1655, Admiral William Penn and his military associate Robert Venables, sent by Oliver Cromwell with a force to attempt to conquer Hispañiola for England, directed their course to Jamaica, where they arrived in May 1655. By October 1655, the Spanish blacks had freed themselves from their masters, and were murdering any of the English rambling about the country who fell into their hands. By the latter part of 1658, however, the English had completely defeated the Spanish in Jamaica. After this defeat, the Spanish made no effort of any consequence to reclaim Jamaica.

When the English took Jamaica, they inherited, along with its native products, such Spanish introductions as sugarcane, bananas, plantain, oranges, limes, ginger, and European vegetables of different descriptions.

The general treatment of the Negroes in the British West Indies was mild, temperate, and indulgent. Instances of cruelty were not only rare, but were always universally reprobated when discovered and—when legally proved—severely punished.

Aboard the British slave ships in the late 1700s, the Negro slaves were cared for quite well, for a healthy slave was a sold slave. At daybreak, they were given water to wash their hands and faces, after which they were given a morning meal. According to the country whence they came, this meal would consist of either imported or cultivated Indian corn, or rice or yams. The slaves were constantly and regularly made to bathe with salt water. Their evening meal varied, consisting sometimes of food to which they had been accustomed in Africa, such as yams or rice, and at other times of provisions brought from Europe, such as dried beans, peas, wheat, shelled barley, or biscuits. All of these were mixed with a sauce made from meat or fish, or with palm oil, a constant and desirable element in African cookery. At each meal the slaves were permitted as much as they could eat, and had likewise a sufficiency of fresh water, unless, during an uncommonly long voyage, the allowance had to be rationed for the sake of preservation.

When a ship touched at any place in her voyage, as frequently happened, such refreshment as the country afforded, like coconuts, oranges, limes, and other fruits, with vegetables of every sort, were distributed among the Negroes, and refreshments of the same kind were freely allowed them at the place of their destination, between the days of their arrival and the time of their sale.

On the sugar plantations the Negroes were divided into three sets or classes, usually called gangs. The first consisted of the healthiest and most robust men and women, whose chief business, out of season, was to clean, hole, and plant the ground, and in crop time, to cut the sugarcane, feed the mills, and attend to the manufacture of sugar. The second gang was composed of boys and girls and of women well into the late stages of pregnancy, whose chief employment was weeding the sugarcane and engaging in other light work adapted to their strength and condition. The third set consisted of very young children, attended by an old woman, who were to gather greens for the pigs and sheep, weed the gardens, or engage in some gentle exercise, merely to preserve them from the habits of idleness.

A slave's day began early. By eight in the morning breakfast was brought to the fields. Prepared by slave women whose sole employment was to act as the cooks for the rest, this meal commonly consisted of boiled yams, eddoes (taroes), okra, calalu, and plantain, or as many of these vegetables as they could produce. These were seasoned with salt and cayenne pepper. At noon, the slaves came home from the fields to prepare their own midday meal and to rest until two in the afternoon; they then worked until sunset.

A practice that prevailed in Jamaica was that of giving the Negroes land to cultivate; they were expected to maintain themselves with the produce of these lands. This custom proved to be both judicious and beneficial.

Natural Diet and Folk Remedies

The agricultural practices of the slaves were not, however, characterized by prudence, because they trusted more in plantains, corn, and other vegetables that were likely to be destroyed by storms than in what might be called ground provisions, such as yams, eddoes, potatoes, cassava, and other esculent roots, all which were out of the reach of hurricanes.

The slaves' houses were some distance from those of their masters and consisted of small, oblong, thatched huts in which they kept all their movables or goods. In each house there was generally a mat to lie on, an earthen pot to boil food in, and a calabash or two to serve as cup and spoon.

The Negroes, although hard-worked, would dance and sing at night and on holidays. They had several sorts of instruments resembling lutes, made of small gourds fitted with necks and strung with horse hairs or peeled stalks of climbing plants or vines. These instruments were sometimes made of hollow timber, covered with parchment or other wetted skin, with a bow for the neck and the strings tied longer or shorter so that the sounds could be varied.

The slaves' method of curing ailments usually consisted of cupping with a calabash on the pained place. First the calabash was applied hot, with some chips or other combustible material burning in it. The calabash was then pulled off the place, which was cut with scarifications. The cupping glass, or calabash, was then applied again.

The slaves used very few decoctions of herbs, no distillations, and no infusions, but usually took the herbs in substance. For instance, in the treatment of venereal disease, they would sometimes grind the roots of the fingrigo and of the lime tree between two stones, stir the mixture in lime juice until it became thick, and make the patient drink the concoction twice a day.

Bathing was done frequently by the slaves. They would boil hay leaves, wild sage, and other herbs in water, then tie the boiled plants together and dip them into a decoction, which they would sprinkle over their bodies.

In Barbados, there were three classes of men—masters, servants, and slaves. The slaves and their posterity, being subject to their masters forever, were kept and preserved with greater care than the servants, who according to the laws of the island were indentured for only five years. The servants had the worst life, for they were put to very hard labor, were ill-housed, and were supplied with a meager diet.

When they first came to the island, the planters themselves didn't consume meat more than twice a week, and for the rest of the week ate potatoes, loblolly (a thick gruel), and bonavist (hyacinth) beans. The servants had no meat at all, unless an ox died; they then feasted as long as it lasted. Until their plantain groves were mature enough to produce fruit, the slaves were fed the same kind of food—mostly bonavist beans, loblolly, and some toasted ears of maize. Such food (especially the loblolly) gave them a desire for something different, but when they had enough plantains, they never complained, for this was one of their favorite food staples.

Their manner of dressing and eating the plantains has best been described by R. Ligon in *A True and Exact History of the Island of Barbados* (London: 1673) in these terms:

'Tis gathered for them (somewhat before it is ripe, for so they desire to have it) upon Saturday, by a keeper of the plantain grove; who is an able Negro, and knows well the numbers of those that are to be fed with this fruit. And he gathers and lays them all together; till they fetch them away, which is about five o'clock in the afternoon. For on that day they break off work sooner by an hour: partly for this purpose, and partly for the fire in the furnaces is to be put out and the engine and the rooms made clean. Besides they are to wash, shave, and trim themselves against Sunday. But 'tis a lovely sight to see a hundred handsome Negroes, men and women, with every one a grass-green bunch of these fruits on their heads, every bunch twice as big as their heads, all coming in a train one after another, the black and green becoming one another. Having brought the fruit home to their own houses, and pulling off the skin of so much as they will use, they boil it in water, making it into balls, and so they eat it. One bunch a week is a Negroe's allowance. To this, no bread, no drink, but water. Their lodging at night a mere board, with nothing under, nor a top of them. They are happy people, whom so little contents. Very good servants, if they are not spoiled by the English.

On Sunday they rest, and have the whole day at their pleasure. And most of them use it as a day of rest and pleasure. But some of them who will make benefit of the day's liberty, go where the mangrove trees grow, and gather the bark of which they make ropes, which they truck away for other commodities, as shirts and drawers.

When they are sick, there are two remedies that cure them. The one [is] an outward [kind], the other an inward medicine. The outward medicine is a thing they call negro-oyle, and 'tis made of Barbary, yellow it is as beeswax, but soft as butter. When they feel themselves ill, they call for some of that, and anoint their bodies, as their breasts, bellies, and sides, and [in just] two days they are perfectly well. But this does the greatest cures upon such, as have bruises or strains in their bodies. The inward medicine is taken, when they find any weakness or decay in their spirits and stomachs, and then a dram or two of kill-devil revives and comforts them much.

The black races of the West Indies during the slavery era, as well as their habits, form a subject of great interest, which has been explored at greater length elsewhere in other history books and sociological works. Gathered as the black peoples were from numerous tribes of Africa, and settled as they were on different islands, they naturally showed not only differences in inherited qualities but also in those habits that they acquired from different masters. Thus, there were British, French, Danish, Irish, Scotch, and Dutch Negroes on the various islands.

Blacks Introduced into North America

Negroes were brought to North America as early as the year 1502. In 1511 they were acclaimed by the Spanish as being more robust and hardy, more capable of enduring fatigue, and more patient under servitude than the original aborigines (American Indians) themselves. The labor of one Negro was valued as equal to that of four Indians. Charles V, in 1517, granted the Spanish merchants the privilege of introducing 4,000 Africans to the Spanish colonies. Queen Elizabeth, in 1562, through her own agent, Sir John Hawkins, engaged in a lucrative African slave trade with these colonists. A Dutch vessel, in 1619, sold part of her cargo of Africans to the British colonists on the James River in Virginia.

The Negroes were brought from the whole western coast of Africa, between the Sahara and the Cape of Good Hope (Kaffraria). There is no record of their lineage. A single ship would bring emigrants of different nations, drawn from places a thousand miles apart in Africa. They came as strangers to each other; they brought no common language, no established customs, no common worship, and no nationality. The admixture of diverse people thus inaugurated was further increased by the numerous and widely remote settlements in North America among which the Negro immigrants were distributed. Never in the same space of time were any people so rudely mixed, shaken together, and sifted out as were these people.

The want of labor to help fell the forests and to clear and cultivate the fields for the needed harvests was a perplexing and vital question in the seventeenth-century colony of Virginia. Indentured servants of both sexes were shipped from England for this purpose. This help was only temporary as indentured service was limited to just a few years at most. At the expiration of his term an indentured servant was given a certain number of acres of land for his own use, thus becoming a master who would himself require hired labor, thereby adding further to the problem that the original introduction of indentured labor into Virginia was intended to settle.

In April 1607 the first North American colony was settled. And in August 1619 an ominous sign appeared on the soil of North America—the African slave. John Rolfe, then at Jamestown, declared thusly: "To begin with, this year, 1619, about the last of August, came in a Dutch man-of-war that sold us twenty negars." The first Assembly had met in July. Thus, free government and African slavery were introduced into America nearly at the same moment. According to J. E. Cooke in his *Virginia, A History of the People* (Boston: Houghton, Mifflin, and Co., 1884), from which this data has been extracted, this "man-of-war" was a pirate ship—a class of vessels common in those days—manned in part by Englishmen. A Captain Samuel Argall, lieutenant-governor of Virginia from 1617 to 1619, was greatly interested in the adventure of shipping slaves to Virginia.

About two months before the first cargo of slaves reached Jamestown, the people of the colony were granted the right of suffrage, for the first time in the New World, through the election of a House of Burgesses. Thus, while the white man in Virginia was enjoying his first rights there as a freeman, the Negro was offered to him as a slave, and was accepted as a godsend. Whether the introduction of slavery was indeed a godsend to Virginia has, however, long been a moot question.

At the time of the introduction of slavery into Virginia, the colony was confined mainly to small settlements along the banks of the James River. The slaves helped to fell the primeval forests to make a passage for their masters' vehicles through the dense woods. Both slave and master shared the dangers and privations of the early life in the wilderness. The black slave accepted the ill luck, or the good luck, that came to the pioneer and was generally treated fairly in all things but his freedom. His lot was frequently a happier one than that of many of the white indentured servants in whom their masters had no pecuniary interest beyond the cost of their transportation to the colony. Very many of these were forced to perform harder tasks than befell the slaves.

The planter regarded his servants—the term "slaves" was rarely used—simply as laborers and domestic attendants who produced his crops and waited upon him. In return, he was to supply them with the necessities of life; there was a well-grounded convention that slaves were a costly luxury. The possession of African slaves, like the system of indentured servitude, was in the eighteenth century a feature of the entire American society, not only of the South. There was little prejudice to speak of against slavery in either the North or the South in those very early years. The predominance of the blacks in the

South was the result largely of climatic conditions. The number of African slaves in North America in 1756, the generation preceding the American Revolution, was almost 300,000; of these some 120,000 were in Virginia, and the rest, about 172,000, were scattered from New England to Georgia. These classes were uniformly treated.

According to Cooke: "The planters readily purchased them to cultivate tobacco; they were scattered among the plantations; and from this small nucleus widened, year by year, the great African shadow, out of which were to issue the lightning and thunder of the future."

During the long period of more than 300 years, from the time the first slaves were introduced by the Spanish to work the mines in Hispañiola to the abolition of Negro slavery by the United States of America, millions of Africans were brought to the New World. These slaves, whether in the West Indies or in the different American colonies, were introduced to the plants of their new country. In the process of adapting to his new surroundings, the African slave unconsciously laid the foundation for twenty-first-century knowledge about the uses of plants, from food to medicine.

Valuable Plants Introduced by the Slaves

One of the natural consequences that followed the beginning of the exploration of the West African coast by the Portuguese after 1492 was their acceptance of slavery, soon to be followed by an active participation in what may be called the lucrative slave trade between the coasts of western Africa and eastern South America.

Indeed, the decade that followed 1492 was one of the most important periods in the documentation of the man-made dispersal of plant materials and products. There is hardly any question that such staple food plants as the yam (*Dioscorea*), the cassava (*Manihot*), maize (*Zea*), the banana and its related plantain species (*Musa*), and sorghum (*Sorghum*), to mention only a few, owe their existence on both sides of the Atlantic to the ever-sailing, fully ladened slave ships of old.

The following enumeration is limited entirely to the plants that accompanied the Negro slaves on their journey into the unknown.

PEANUT *(Arachis hypogaea).*   "The fruit, which are called by seamen earth-nuts, are brought from Guinea in the negroes ships, to feed the negroes withal in their voyages from Guinea to Jamaica," reported H. Sloane in his *Natural History of Jamaica* (London: 1707–25; 1:184). H. Barnham, in his *Hortus Americanus* (Kingston, Jamaica: Alexander-Aikman, 1794; p. 145), noted this: "The first time I ever saw one of these growing was in a negro's plantation, who affirmed, that they grew in great plenty in their own country; and now they grow here [in Jamaica]."

AKEE *(Blighia sapida).*   "This grand and magnificent vegetable has been brought to Jamaica by a slave ship coming from the coast of Guinea; it is perfectly naturalized," wrote F. R. Tussac in his *Flore des Antilles* (Paris: 1808–27; 2:66).

PIGEON PEA *(Cajanus cajan).*   Tussac stated this in his large multivolumed work (4:95): "The cytisus of the Indies or Angola pea, has been brought from Africa by the Negroes, who have introduced them to the Antilles; there it has been so well naturalized that it passes for being native, which I do not believe, having found it only on cultivated land. This interesting shrub, producing flowers and fruits during nine months of the year has the double advantage to ornate the sides of the alleys separating the pieces of sugarcane, and to furnish the whites and Negroes a healthy and agreeable nourishment."

MARIJUANA *(Cannabis sativa).*   R. P. Walton wrote this interesting background relative to one of America's most medically useful but still highly illegal drugs in his fascinating study *Marihuana: America's New Drug Problem* (New York City: J. B. Lippincott Co., 1938; p. 24): "The hemp plant reputedly was introduced into Chile by the Spaniards about 1545. This was mainly or solely for the purposes of fiber production. The vice seems to have migrated with African slaves at some undetermined date. This general opinion is often cited and, among other evidence, it is supported by similarity in the names used in both places. Diamba and riamba are terms used by West African negroes, and the same terms are used in Brazil. Lucena and also Doria say that the 'maconha' smoked in Brazil is an African variety of cannabis. Iglesias reported in 1918 that the practice was extremely prevalent in Brazil and said that it was cultivated chiefly in certain regions in the northern part where it was smoked in special pipes which passed the smoke through water or that it was sometimes smoked in the form of a cigarette or cigar."

SENNA *(Cassia italica).* "The Jamaican senna, a substitute for the official senna is said to have been introduced by a slave during the seventeenth century. The product is still in use," observed F. F. Cassidy and R. B. Le Page in their *Dictionary of Jamaican English* (Cambridge, England: Cambridge University Press, 1967; p. 242).

BISSY NUT TREE/KOLA NUT *(Cola acuminata).* "The seed brought in a Guinea ship from that country, was here planted by Mr. Goffee in Colonel Bourder's plantation beyond Guanoboa. It is called bichy by the Coromantyn Negroes, and is both eaten and used for physic in pains of the belly," noted Sloane (2:61).

The kola nut, as it has come to be popularly known in the food, beverage, and herbal industries, is primarily utilized for its high caffeine content (usually 1.5 to 2 percent). It is a stimulant to the central nervous system and has been used in certain herbal preparations in treating obesity, fatigue, migraine, neuralgia, diarrhea, and other conditions. Kola extracts are widely used as a flavoring agent in cola drinks. Other food products in which kola extracts are used are alcoholic beverages, frozen dairy desserts, candy, baked goods, and gelatins and puddings. The kola nut was the subject of a German therapeutic monograph as an analeptic for use in mental and physical fatigue. (See Monograph *Colae semen*, in *Bundesanzeiger,* no. 127, July 12, 1991.)

MAROON CUCUMBER/WEST INDIAN GHERKIN *(Cucumis anguria).* According to A. De Candolle in his *Origin of*

Cultivated Plants (London: Trench and Co., 1884; p. 268): "M. Naudin was the first to point out that all the other species of *Cucumis* are of the Old World, and principally Africa. He wondered whether this one had not been introduced into America by the Negroes, like many other plants which have become naturalized. However, unable to find any similar African plant, he adopted the general opinion. Sir Joseph Hooker, on the contrary, is inclined to believe that *C. anguria* is a cultivated and modified form of some African species nearly allied to *C. prophetarum* and *C. figarei*, although these are perennial. In favor of this hypothesis, I may add: (1) the name maroon cucumber, given in the French West Indies Islands, indicates a plant which has become wild, for this is the meaning of the word maroon as applied to the Negroes; (2) its extended area in America from Brazil to the West Indies, always along the coast where the slave trade was most brisk, seems to be a proof of foreign origin."

YAM BACARA *(Dioscorea alata).*   About this edible food staple, Tussac (4:82) wrote as follows: "Under the plants of major importance which have been introduced in the Antilles and which are naturalized, the yam must always rank first; the genus of this plant is native of the country, but the kind I am going to describe, like the prickly yam or yam of Guinea, have been brought from Africa by the Negroes.

"The yams are eaten in several manners: the one used mostly by the wealthy colonists, is to cook them with a little salt, and sometimes with nearly ripe bananas; this is a basic dish, like the cooked beef in France. The Negroes eat them in the same manner, and it is eaten with their calalou. Many Americans, especially in Jamaica, prefer the yam to bread. The root of the yam is suitable for alcoholic fermentation, and one can produce a kind of beer with it. The yam is an important commercial subject for the free Negroes and the slaves, who cultivate them in their gardens, sell them at the markets found on Sundays in all villages of the country."

YELLOW YAM *(Dioscorea cayanensis).*   Piso and Marcgrave in their fascinating *Historiae Naturalis Brasiliae* (1648) imply that the yellow yam, although having originated somewhere in Southeast Asia, probably reached Brazil via Africa due to such common names as inhame de S. Thome, cara brasiliensibus, inhame, camaranbaya, and quingumbo. It is from this widely popular tuber vegetable that the early black slaves obtained much of their vitamins A and C.

AFRICAN OIL PALM *(Elaeis guineensis).* W. Wright, in his article, "An Account of the Medicinal Plants Growing in Jamaica," which appeared in the *London Medical Journal* (3[3]:293; 1787) commented on this plant as follows: "This was originally brought from Guinea by the Negroes. The trunk is straight, and guarded by numerous long spines, or needles. The fruit is triangular, yellow, and as big as a plum. The nut, or kernel, by decoction, yields the oleum palmae of the shops."

CALABASH NUTMEG *(Monodora myristica).* A.H.R. Grisebach in his *Flora of the British West Indies* (London: Lovell Reeve and Co., 1859–64; p. 8) gave this background history: "Formerly introduced into Jamaica, the specimens in the Hookerian Herbarium, dating from 1830, but now perhaps extinct. Mr. March states in a letter, that the two trees recorded in Macfadyen's Flora, have been lost, but that it may be found still at the old Botanic Garden, S. Andrew's, where it was at one time known to exist.

"R. Brown was of the opinion that the Calabash Nutmeg might have been introduced by the Negroes from the west coast of Africa. And Sir W. Hooker led me to inquire whether the *Xylopia undulata* of Palisot de Beauvois's *Flore d'Oware* (*Habzelia* a. D.C.) was not the same plant.

"The author states that he observed the fruits in the markets of the Guinea coast, and that afterward the tree flowering and bearing fruits of a former year, when he travelled in the interior of Ware, seventy or eighty leagues from the coast. Now the fruit which he figures, though indeed in connection with the flowering branch, is not a remnant of a former year, but a well-developed, just ripe system of carpids, quite similar to those of *Habzelia aethiopica,* which are known to have been common in the African market."

BROAD BEAN *(Phaseolus lunatus)*.   C. Bryant claimed in his *Flora Diaetetica: or History of Esculent Plants* (London: 1783; p. 307) the following origin for this useful plant: "The common broad bean is a native of Egypt, and like the pea is now run into many varieties, which have their distinguishing appellations among the gardeners. The only variety taken notice of by Linneaus is the horsebean, and even this now is run into many variations. These are not eaten in England, but our merchants ship them for Africa, where they are brought for the slaves in their voyage to the West Indies."

SESAME SEED *(Sesamum indicum)*.   Bryant wrote this about sesame seed and sesame oil in particular: "This is an annual, and grows naturally in the island of Ceylon, and on the coast of Malabar. This plant is not only cultivated in Asia, but also in Africa, and from the latter the Negroes have carried it to South Carolina, where they raise large quantities of it, being very fond of the seeds, and make soups and puddings of them, as with rice and millet. They parch them over the fire, and with other ingredients stew them into a hearty food. The seed in Carolina is called 'oily grain' it yielding oil very copiously. This when first drawn has a warm, pungent taste, and is otherwise not palatable. But after being kept a year or two, the disagreeableness goes off, and it becomes mild and pleasant, is then used in their salads, and for all purposes of olive oil."

SORGHUM *(Sorghum vulgare)*.   M. Catesby wrote the following about this bunched guinea corn or type of millet in *The Natural History of Carolina, Florida, and the Bahama Islands* (London: 1754; I:xviii): "Little of this grain is propagated, and that chiefly by Negroes, who make bread of it, and boil it in like manner of furmety. Its chief use is for feeding fowls, for which the smallness of the grain adapts it. It was first introduced from Africa by the Negroes."

And Bryant (p. 336) added this bit of information: "[Sorghum is] native [to] India, and [is] cultivated in Africa under the name of Guinea corn. . . . The grain is there made into bread, and is otherwise used, and is deemed wholesome food. From Africa the Negroes carried them to the West Indies, where they are both sown for their use, and each slave is generally allowed from a pint to a quart per day."

SURINAM POISON *(Tephorsia sinapou).* Tussac (1:45) wrote about this stupefying herb root as follows: "This plant was, they say, brought from Africa to the Antilles by the Negroes. It was perhaps too well naturalized there, because of the way the creoles sometimes abused its bad qualities. The roots, which have a nauseating odor, are believed in the country to be extremely antiseptic. A reliable source assured me that a chronic sore was cured by the repeated application of a decoction made of these roots; taken internally, others regard it as a poison. The Negroes use the leaves of this plant, pounded between two stones to make a paste, to paralyze or even kill the fish in the rivers; they mix this kind of paste with cassava. A fish when killed this way, does no harm to whoever eats it."

BLACK-EYED PEAS *(Vigna unguiculata).* R. W. Schery stated in his *Plants for Man* (New York: Prentice Hall, Inc., 1952; p. 404): " 'Peas' in the Deep South of the United States invariably means cowpeas or black-eyed peas. . . . Actually this species is more related to beans than to peas. It was introduced into the West Indies from central Africa, and thence into the Carolinas before the early 1700's. Today it is perhaps more grown as a green manure and forage plant than for the black-eyed peas dishes omnipresent in the south."

Medicinal Plants Employed by Slaves in the West Indies and Colonial America

The Negro slaves were essentially primitive men with a belief that diseases were due to the presence of evil spirits in the body, much as the ancient civilizations did and which has already been mentioned in the opening chapters of this text.

The slaves were equally convinced that every disease could be cured through the use of disagreeable or often poisonous substances that would make the body an unpleasant place for the disembodied spirits to want to inhabit. Since the Negro slave had brought with him an intimate knowledge of nature, he began his new life in the Americas using the process of trial and error to find suitable substitutes for the plants he had used in his homeland. His whole endeavor was deeply rooted in superstition and pure speculation. Yet through these avenues he found an array of plants that he learned to use with success in his everyday life.

I've taken the liberty to arrange the following data alphabetically, using the Latin binomials for each entry, followed by their common names. The sources used for the interesting information given here have already been cited in the previous section; therefore, it won't be necessary to repeat them here.

Many of these remedies, while quite old, are still very efficacious and can be used with reasonable safety and common sense.

OKRA *(Abelmoschus esculentus).*   This vegetable is believed to have originated in the northeastern part of the African continent and grows wild in upper Egypt and in Libya. It was brought to the Americas in the 1600s by black slaves and has found itself exceptionally popular in the unique Creole and Cajun cookery styles indigenous to Louisiana.

Okra pods were and still are boiled when young and tender to make a type of slimy broth, which is then administered to invalids. Being of a strong lubricative texture and high in protein content, okra broth in this form affords a very agreeable nutritious food to help sick and bedridden folks recuperate more rapidly from their ailments.

GREAT MACKAW TREE *(Acrocomia sclerocarpa).*   The slaves of the Americas utilized the oil of the fruit of this tree as an emollient for aching bones, stiff joints, and sore muscles; they liberally applied it externally and thoroughly massaged it into the skin for great relief. The nut inside the fruit was sometimes skillfully carved by the Negroes for relaxation and then buffed to a very high polish afterward.

ANTILLES AGAVE *(Agave antillarum).*   The slaves of the Antilles once used an alcoholic tincture of this as an effective detergent for the cure of skin ulcers and gangrene. The Negroes created an embrocation of the following ointment: One pound of the juice of the agave was mixed with 8 ounces of sugared orange juice, then 8 ounces of *Guaiacum officinale* and 8 ounces of hog's lard were added. M. E. Descourtilz, from whom this data came, declared in his *Flore Pittoresque et Mèdical Des Antilles* (Paris: 1833; 4:243) that "this makes [a] great cure without fail!"

Another species of agave (*Agave virginica*) has been used as a reliable remedy for flatulence and stomach colic in the Deep South. It was used on St. John's Island in South Carolina for treating rattlesnake bite.

COMMON ONION *(Allium cepa).*   In 1792 an elderly Negro man aged 72 was cured of kidney stones by taking the expelled juice of red onions along with horsemint. He took a stronger than usual decoction of the latter on account of the herb being dry. In about a week's time the stones began to dissolve of their own accord. The cure was completed in about six months' time. This discovery was made by another Negro slave in Virginia, who treated his white master with it, thereby obtaining his freedom on account of its success.

CASHEW *(Anacardium occidentale).*   In olden times many Negroes suffered from dropsy. But if they were allowed to eat plentifully of the roasted kernels of cashew nuts, they would soon recover from their edemas.

PINEAPPLE *(Ananas comosus).*   Slaves often praised the virtues of this humble fruit for its ability to cure atonic ulcers and for correcting digestive upset. An old Negro remedy from those times called for 2 ounces of pineapple juice, 2 ounces of combined agave and aloe leaves, 1 ounce of balsam of sugar, the yolk of one egg, and a little rum. Everything was mixed together and a little bit taken with a meal to prevent indigestion.

RATTLESNAKE'S MASTER *(Aralia spinosa).*   In South Carolina this plant was once considered "the rattlesnake's master par excellence" with slaves. The fresh root is taken internally, as well as applied in powdered form externally to the wounded part itself.

JACK IN THE PULPIT *(Arisaema triphyllum)*.   In the *Journal of Benjamin Smith Barton on a Visit to Virginia in 1802* (1938:1:110) is found this short anecdote: "[It] was related to me the case of a negro-man, who was entirely cured of a consumption of his lungs, by giving him to drink, for a considerable time, milk in which was boiled the root of the Indian turnip *Arum triphyllum*. The milk was strongly impregnated with the acrimony of the root."

SNAKEROOT *(Aristolochia serpentaria)*.   The Negroes of South Carolina often made much use of this valuable plant, especially when any of them were in the low stages of pneumonia, to which they were particularly susceptible. The dose of the powdered root was 10 to 30 grains; of the infusion of 1 ounce of root to 1 pint of boiling water, about 2 ounces of liquid were used as the occasion required. Its effects were increased by combining it with camphor.

WILD IPECACUHANA *(Ascelpias curassavica)*.   This plant is common throughout Jamaica. Thomas Nicol, an early practitioner there in 1814, told of its wonderful and amazing styptic virtues. He recalled an incident that involved a certain mule that had met with some kind of violent accident, resulting in a serious thigh wound from which the blood issued in great quantities. A Negro who happened to be standing nearby spotted some of this wild ipecac, and grabbing a handful of its blossoms and leaves, bruised them well between his big hands and then applied the plant matter directly to the open wound. The bleeding "stopped instantaneously," according to reliable eyewitnesses who were there at the time. Dr. Nicol employs wild ipecac and cayenne pepper together for stopping even the most serious hemorrhaging in humans.

BROOM WEED *(Baccharis scoparia)*.   In olden times slave women would sometimes wash their children in a bath of this herb if their skin happened to be scabby or mangy-looking. It would thoroughly cleanse them and make them thrive again.

HOG DOCTOR TREE *(Bursera simaruba/Terebinthus sima–*
ruba). Old Negro slaves would use the balsam of this plant as a
dressing for sordid ulcers. The tincture proved very useful for moder-
ating the excessive flow of certain leuchorrheas (vaginal discharge of
pus or mucus), the spitting up of blood, and hemorrhages. In other
cases, the tincture strengthened the stomach, the heart, and the brain
by accelerating blood circulation. Those who suffered from consumption of the lungs were give up to 10 drops in a glass of milk. Several
asthmatics who made use of this tincture soon found themselves totally cured of their ailment.

BASTARD MAMEE *(Calophyllum calaba).* H. Barham reported in his *Hortus Americanus* (Kingston, Jamaica: Alexander-
Aikman, 1794; p. 18): "I once had a green balsam presented to me,
brought from the Spaniards, of a very fine green, clear, and pleasant
smell, which they said was the finest balsam in the world for green
wounds. But they could not tell me from what tree it came. Some time
after this, a negro brought me of the same sort of balsam, both in
color and smell, which he got from one of these trees. I found it to be
an excellent balsam. For, I melt and pour it into a green or fresh in-
cised wound and it would heal up in [just] one or two dressings."

HORSE BEAN/OVERLOOK *(Canavalia ensiformis).* Not
all plants were employed for nutritive or remedial purposes; some
such as this were used purely for superstitious reasons, as author J.
Macfadyen reported in his *Flora of Jamaica* (London: Longmens
Green, 1837; 1:179): "[It] was commonly planted by Jamaican negroes, along the margin of their provision grounds, from a superstitious notion, probably of African origin, very generally entertained,
that the Overlook fulfills the parts of a watchman. And from some
dreaded or awful power ascribed to it by them, protects their provisions from plunder by midnight thieves. Even the better informed
among them continue to adopt this practice, although they may not
place much confidence in any particular influence which this humble
plant is presumed to exercise, either in preventing theft outright or
else in punishing the perpetrators thereof when the crime has been
committed."

GUINEA BIRD PEPPER/CAYENNE PEPPER *(Capsicum annuum).* Slaves in the United States came to rely upon this spice for medicinal reasons, besides the usual culinary purposes for which it was chiefly employed. It was particularly useful for a condition formerly known as cachexia. This was a general weight loss and wasting occurrence in the course of an existing chronic disease or due to some kind of emotional upset. "Cachexia africana" was then a common affliction among a number of slaves working on plantations throughout the South; it resulted in a dramatic fall of body temperature, severe electrolyte imbalance, and hypoglycemia; and unless immediately attended to would usually result in coma and death. The slaves discovered that cayenne pepper administered in a warm liquid broth of some kind could reverse most of these symptoms within an hour or so. It was also very efficacious in the treatment of low blood pressure, poor circulation, coldness in the lower extremities, and diabetes. And when some powdered red pepper was sprinkled on an external hemorrhage of some kind, the bleeding would cease almost immediately.

PAPAYA/PAPAW *(Carica papaya).* The Negroes of the Antilles were quite superstitious with regard to the presumed good and bad qualities of certain trees. They presumed that papaya trees rendered the air healthy and would therefore plant them near their homes. The blossoms are extremely odoriferous and the trunks so succulent and fast-growing that the slaves probably thought the trees assisted in draining the soil of superfluous moisture wherever they happened to be planted. The Negroes sincerely believed that the trees' wonderfully aromatic virtues could correct the "bad" air caused by invisible and malovent spirits, thereby dispelling disease and airborne sicknesses.

They gave the fruit to invalids to help them recuperate from long-term illnesses and bed confinement. They frequently placed ripe papaya slices directly on open wounds, skin sores, and bed sores to help them clear up and heal more rapidly. Ripe papaya fruit was also consumed to eliminate belly ache caused by overeating or eating too much hog meat.

RINGWORM BUSH *(Cassia alata).*   Tetters or ringworm was quite common among the early black slaves in Jamaica, and among the Spaniards in America it was an almost daily occurrence. In fact, this complaint was so universal throughout the Americas that the skin of many of those severely afflicted with it looked almost leprous. The hapless victims suffered from intolerable itching or painful skin ulcers and were forever scratching themselves to obtain some measure of relief. A poultice of the flowers of this bush was of great service, as were sulphur-containing applications. But in the more advanced stages of this disease, remedies containing liquid mercury and decoctions of certain wood barks were the only chance for a cure.

Another species of cassia *(Cassia chamaecrista)* was an effective antidote against certain types of subtlely administered poisons. A handful of the washed roots were boiled in 3 pints of water for an hour, strained, sweetened, and then used as a common drink at the rate of 3 quarts in 24 hours, during which time the deleterious effects of the poison would usually pass.

Another kind of cassia or senna *(Cassia occidentalis)* was employed by Jamaican Negroes in the preparation of their baths and for fomentation purposes. The leaves would also be smeared with a little candle grease and then applied to skin sores as an effective substitute for adhesive plaster.

A decoction of the leaves was used against inflammations of the anus and the ulcerations produced by the presence of insects that the Portuguese called Bicho del cu. This decoction was also successfully prescribed for erysipelas of the legs.

The root of the species known as *Cassia viminea* or attoo was used by the Jamaican Negroes as a type of natural toothbrush to cleanse their teeth. They would also grind it up and mix the powder with some water to make a paste that they would then plaster all over the body during periods of fever, headaches, or colic.

SNAKEWOOD/TRUMPET TREE *(Cecropia peltata).*   Slaves in the Americas would use the white, fat, and juicy pith of the hollows on top of these trees, as well as their young leaves, to wash their wounds and old sores. They used the burnt bark and leaf ashes to cure their dropsy by mixing in some water and consuming it. The tree sap that flowed from gashes made in the trunk with a machete was often collected and used to dress wounds. The inner layer of the trunk bark is quite astringent and was used for healing venereal diseases.

WILD COTTON TREE *(Ceiba pentandra).*   The young and tender tree leaves are quite mucilaginous and formed an important food source for many Negroes when boiled in cast-iron pots.

But the tree itself was once highly venerated by all slaves in the tropical Americas, as both Stedman and Macfadyen have pointed out in their respective works. "All negroes believe in the being of a God, upon whose goodness they rely, and whose power they adore," wrote Stedman (2:271). "They have no fear of death, and never taste food without offering a libation of some kind. In the rivers of Gambia and Senegal they are mostly Mahometans. But generally the worship and religious ceremonies of the Africans vary, as to the numberless super-stitious practices of all savages, and indeed of too many Europeans.

"Perceiving that it was their custom to bring their offerings to the wild cotton tree, I enquired of an old negro, why they paid such par-ticular reverence and veneration to this growing piece of timber. 'This proceeds (said he) massera, from the following cause: We have no churches nor places built for public worship (as you have) on the coast of Guinea. And [since] this tree being the largest and most beau-tiful growing here, our people assemble under its branches when they are to be instructed. And are defended by it from the heavy rains and scorching sun. Under this tree our gadoman, or priest, delivers his lec-tures; and for this reason our common people have so much veneration for it, that they will not cut it down upon any account whatever.'"

Macfadyen noted this: "Even the untutored children of Africa are so struck with the majesty of its appearance, that they designate it the God-tree, and account it sacrilege to injure it with an axe. So that, not infrequently, not even the fear of punishment will induce them to cut it down. Even in a state of decay, it is [still] an object of their super-stitious fears; they regard it as consecrated to spirits, whose favor they seek to conciliate by offerings placed at its base."

LIME *(Citrus aurantifolia).* Since there are so many varied and interesting medicinal uses for this particular citrus fruit, I will cite the different sources quoted from in passing.

W. Smith in his classic study *A Natural History of Nevis, and the Rest of the English Leeward Charibee Islands in America* (Cambridge, England: 1745; p. 232) related the following episode: "My servant man Oxford, had once on a sudden, got a cerbouga, (that is to say, a fleshy substance, not unlike a wart) growing in the middle of the bottom of his right foot, that was about the size of a common nutmeg, and quite lamed him up. [But] he was cured in the following manner. An old experienced mulatto woman, took a good sharp penknife and cut it, till it bled; then she seared it with a red-hot iron, and applied to burn, half of a lime or bastard lemon, which in two or three days time, brought out the whole cerbouga, just like the core of an apple. Oxford was not lame for it above sixteen days and continued to serve me well as a good Negro should."

H. Barnham (cited before) mentioned this about limes: "The negroes and Indians use the root of the tree in venereal cases, and the stalk to clean their teeth with."

Both E. Long in his *History of Jamaica* (London: T. Lowndes, 1774; 3:795) and J. Lunan in his *Hortus Jamaicensis* (Jamaica: St. Jago De La Vega Gazette, 1814; 1:452) both stated the same thing in their respective works, as follows: "The negroes take the young fruit soon after it is formed, or when it is about the size of a small hazelnut, pare off the rind, which they beat into a fine pulp, and with a hair pencil apply it carefully to the lids of sore eyes, for a cure. It is supposed, this rawness of the eye-lid, accompanied with a humour, is generally caused by worms, which lodge in it, and that the application destroys them. This hint is worth a further attention, since the animaleules, if they really lodge there, may be discovered by proper glasses; and hence the knowledge obtained, whether the application would be proper or otherwise."

M.L.P. Du Pratz had a lot to say about the use of limes in his *History of Louisiana, or of the Western parts of Virginia and Carolina* (London: T. Becket, 1774; pp. 378–80): "The negro who taught me these two remedies, observing the great care I took of both the negro men and negro women, taught me likewise the cure of all the distempers to which the women are subject; for the negro women are as liable to diseases as the white women tend to be.

"You must never put an iron instrument into the yaw [a large granulomatous lesion present on the hand, leg, or foot]; such an application would be certain death. In order to open the yaw, you take the iron rust reduced to an impalpable powder, and passed through a fine search. You afterward mix the powder with citrus juice till it be of the consistence of an ointment, which you spread upon a linen cloth greased with hog's grease, or fresh lard without salt, for want of a better. You lay the plaster upon the yaw, and renew it evening and morning, which will open the yaw in a very short time without any incision.

"The opening being once made, you take about the bulk of a goose's egg of hog's lard without salt, in which you incorporate about an ounce of good terebinthine. After which take a quantity of powdered verdigris, and soak it half a day in good vinegar, which you must then pour off gently with all the scrum that floats a top it. Drop a cloth all over with the verdigris that remains, and upon that apply your last ointment. [*Author's note:* Verdigris is the green or greenish-blue deposit formed on copper, brass, or bronze surfaces. It has been a common medicinal agent since ancient times.]

"All these operations are to be performed without the assistance of any fire. The whole ointment being well mixed with a spatula, you dress the yaw with it. After that you put your negro in a copious sweat, and he will be cured. Take special care that your surgeon does not use mercurial medicine, as I have seen; for that will occasion the death of the patient, for a good, strong, working negro is hard to replace; therefore, every effort should be made to save him at all costs, as he represents for you a great investment.

"The scurvy is no less to be dreaded than the yaws; nevertheless, you may get the better of it, by adhering exactly to the following prescription: Take some scurvy-grass, for you have plants of it, some ground ivy, called by some St. John's wort, some water-cresses from a spring or brook, and for want of that wild-cresses. Take these three herbs, or the last two, if you have no scurvy-grass; pound them and mix them with citron [lime]-juice, to make of them a soft paste, which the patient must keep upon the gums till they be clean, at all times when he is eating.

"In the meantime he must be suffered to drink nothing but an infusion of the herbs [just] named. You pound two handfuls of them, roots and all, after washing off the earth that may be upon the roots or leaves; to these you join a fresh citron [lime], cut into slices. Having pounded all together, you then steep them in an earthen pan in a pint of pure water of the measure of Paris. After that you add about the size of a walnut of powdered and purified saltpetre. To make it a little relishing to the negro, you add some powdered sugar. After the water has stood one night, you squeeze out the herbs pretty strongly. The whole is performed cold or without fire. Such is the dose for a bottle of water Paris measure; but as the patient ought to drink two pints a day, you may make several pints at a time in the above proportion.

"In these two distempers the patients must be supported with good nourishment, and [made] to sweat copiously. It would be a mistake to think that they ought to be kept to a spare diet; you must give them nourishing food, but a little at a time. A negro can no more than any other person support remedies upon bad food, and still less upon a spare diet. But the quality must be proportioned to the state of the patient, and the nature of the distemper [itself]. Besides, good food makes the best part of the remedy to those who in common are but poorly fed."

Stedman said this about the benefits of limes in his particular work (cited earlier in the text): "The negroes (in Surinam) are very subject to this complaint (swelled foot, a disease called consaca, not unlike our chilblains in Europe, as it occasions a very great itching, particularly between the toes, whence issues a very watery fluid), which they cure by applying the skin of a lemon or lime, made as hot as they can bear it.

"The clabba-yaws, or tubboes, is also a very troublesome and tedious disorder; it occasions painful sores about the feet, mostly in the soles, between the skin and the flesh. The usual remedy in this case is, to burn out the morbid part with a red-hot iron, or cut it out with a lancet; and then warm juice of roasted limes is introduced into the wound, though with great pain yet with great success."

Tussac (cited earlier) added these several tidbits concerning limes: "The fruits of this plant are also used in the hospitals of the natives, for curing or preventing the panaris [a purulent infection or abscess involving the bulbous distal end of a finger]. The negroes smoke it, which means cook them in ashes. They cut the outside and stick their sore finger into the inside, at the highest degree of heat they can take. This remedy is successful very often, either in curing the panaris or in stopping it from spreading. The negro washerwomen [also] use them for cleansing their laundry."

SOUR ORANGE *(Citrus aurantium).*   Stedman wrote this: "The oranges in Surinam are of three different species: the sour, the bitter, and the sweet, all being originally imported from Spain or Portugal. The sour oranges are an excellent cure for sores and running ulcers, so common in this climate, but painful in this operation; for which reason they are only used for the negroes, who it is supposed may bear anything."

And Tussac added this in his monumental work: "The negroes make great usage of the sour oranges, be it raw, be it smoked, which means cooked in the ashes, for dressing old wounds, be it men, be it of horses. Furthermore, this remedy is a strong detergent, it stops vermin from entering the wounds, or kills them."

LEMON *(Citrus limon).*   Descourtilz made this observation in his multivolumed set (cited earlier): "The negroes also praise a remedy which they use for the care of tapeworm: that is a glass of lemon juice in which one has put two inches of ash. The worm dies, but one has to have recourse on purgatives for expelling it."

CLEMATIS *(Clematis dioica).*   Macfadyen listed these medicinal uses for the plant: "The leaves are hot and acrid to taste, and when bruised into a pulp, and applied to the skin, they act as a rubefacient, and even vesicate (blister). An infusion of the bruised leaves and flowers forms a good lotion for the removal of spots and freckles from the skin. And a decoction of the root in sea-water, mixed with wine, is said to act as a powerful purge in hydropic cases."

BASTARD MUSTARD *(Cleome gynandra).*   The juice of this plant, when mixed with sweet oil, was looked upon to be a sovereign remedy against pain in the ear if poured into it while still warm. Lunan (1:67; cited earlier) gave this case study "in confirmation of the above virtue in this plant of curing pains in the ears": "A gentleman of St. Elizabeth's informed me, that for some years he had been at times afflicted with violent pains in his left ear, so that at last he could hardly hear on that side. He had little or no wax at any time in it. [He] sometimes felt such an uneasy sensation, as one perceives when a flea or some other small insect gets into one's ear, that in a few days before he saw me he had [actually] pulled a living insect out of it. He said, that when the pain was most raging he had on the advice of a negro woman, taken a leaf of the [bastard mustard] and upon squeezing a few drops of it into his ear, he had been instantaneously relieved from the pain."

COCONUT *(Cocos nucifera).*   Jamaican slaves recommended ground coconut shell taken every morning on an empty stomach in a glass of Medeira wine to regain the strength of the [en]feeble[d]. This preparation, they noted, accelerated blood circulation and was very favorable for the elderly.

BISSY NUT/COLA NUT *(Cola acuminata).*   Guinea negroes used this as a physic for relieving stomach cramps. And Jamaican negroes mixed the ground cola nut with some capsicum for "complaints of the belly."

DOGWOOD *(Cornus florida).*   The old Creole negroes who once inhabited Norfolk, Virginia, in great numbers were in the habit of using dogwood twigs for cleaning their teeth after a meal. Barton attested to the sound dental hygiene that resulted from this common practice: "The striking whiteness of these, which I have frequently observed, is a proof of the efficacy of the practice. The application of the juice of the twigs to the gums, is also useful in preserving them hard and sound."

JERUSALEM ARTICHOKE *(Cynara scolymus).* Great use was made of this vegetable on the plantations in the Deep South as a tonic and diuretic in cases of dropsy. The leaves were steeped in rum for several days and a wine-glassful then taken 3 times a day for this problem with good results.

PERSIMMON *(Diospyros virginiana).* Barton (cited earlier) wrote this in his journal (2:52): "In the course of my journey through Virginia, in the year 1802, I was informed, that the ripe fruit of the persimmon . . . has often been found very useful in the worm-cases of the negro and other children. . . . Perhaps, it operates in this manner solely by the virtue of a laxative property."

PALM OIL *(Elaeis guineensis).* G. Hughes in his book *The Natural History of Barbados* (London: 1750; p. 112) wrote this about palm oil: "The inhabitants of Africa anoint their bodies with it, to supple and relax their stiffened nerves, as well as to prevent a too plentiful perspiration.

"This is so universal a custom, that all slaves, brought now from any part of Africa to this, or any of our neighboring Islands, are always, before they are brought to market to be sold, anointed all over with palm oil, which, for that purpose, is brought from Guiney: being thus anointed, their skins appear sleek and shining."

R. Ligon in his *A True and Exact History of the Island of Barbados* (London: 1673; p. 51) described the use of palm oil by slaves in this interesting manner: "The outward medicine is a thing they call negro-oyle, and 'tis made in Barbary, yellow it is as beeswax, but soft as butter. When they feel themselves ill, they call for some of that, and in two days they are perfectly well [again]. But this does the greatest cures upon such, as have bruises or strains in their bodies."

BONESET *(Eupatorium perfoliatum).* This plant was extensively employed by the Negroes on the cotton and tobacco plantations in South Carolina as a tonic and diaphoretic in colds and fevers, as well as in typhoid pneumonia, which was so prevalent among them in those times.

Descourtilz (3:214) gave additional data concerning boneset: "It seems certain that one can immune oneself against the most venomous snakes, and challenge their bites utilizing the following procedure. The negroes' practice is to make six incisions, two at the feet, two at the hands, and one at each side of the chest, of the wound. One squeezes the sap of the leaves of [boneset], which he [then] pours on the incisions as if he were inoculating for smallpox. After the operation make the patient swallow two spoons of the plant sap. The patient is advised to take the same sap for five or six days. If he neglects to do this several times, the virtue of the sap disappears, and he will need a new inoculation."

FIG *(Ficus indica).* Island Negroes employed fig fruit for expediting recovery from long-term sickness. The figs were sometimes stewed or boiled and then eaten to soften the stools and improve digestion. Fresh fig poultices were used to withdraw purulent matter from lanced boils or sores. They were used both ways (internally as well as externally) to reduce malignant tumors.

COTTON *(Gossypium herbaceum).* The Negroes in the Southern states relied upon cotton root as an effective abortifacient. They would gather sufficient quantities of cotton root, clean it, boil it, and then drink the tea to cause a spontaneous abortion during the first few weeks of pregnancy.

MALLOW *(Hibiscus elatus).* This species is related to okra, with which gumbo is made. The young shoots and leaves of this shrub yield an abundant amount of fine mucilage. They were extensively employed during the several centuries of slavery in the Americas for dysentery. The plant materials would be infused in boiling water and then drunk when warm.

MANCHANEEL *(Hippomane mancinella).* In his insightful book on the history of Barbados, author O. Hughes mentioned this little episode concerning the rather unorthodox use of this volatile herb somewhere in the middle part of the eighteenth century.

"One instance of its malignancy happened about two years ago in Speights-town. A certain slave, conceiving herself injuriously treated, poured into her master's chocolate about a spoonful of this juice. Immediately after he had swallowed it, he felt a violent burning in his throat and stomach. Suspecting he was poisoned, he strove and with good success to vomit. And having taken after this seasonable discharge, a regular emetic, his stomach was, in a great measure, suddenly cleansed of the poison, tho' it cost him a long time to perfect the cure."

SANDBOX TREE *(Hura crepitans).*   Some botanicals, while excellent remedies in their own right, are so powerful that they need to be used judiciously and with great wisdom; if they're not, unhappy consequences may result. Tussac (4:23) reported this: "Here is an incident that I witnessed in Port-au-Prince [Haiti]. A colored woman over many years made an oil from the seeds of the sandbox tree, either to clear herself or to purge her negroes by mitigating this remedy. The day she prepared the oil she left the house for a moment, leaving two negro women inside [who were unacquainted with its effects]. These two unhappy ones dipped cassava into the oil, and when she returned the two negresses were dying without being taken care of by a skillful doctor who knew about the effects of such a poison."

Descourtilz (2:226) informed his readers that "the negroes apply the green leaves of the Hura infused in oil on parts effected by chronic pains."

SPIKENARD *(Hyptis suaveolens).*   In the days of slavery, owners would sometimes give a special decoction made with this plant to their Negroes who suffered from the nasty effects of smallpox or the debilitating condition of heart disease. They would mix lemons, sugar, a little spirit of vitriol, and an oily spirit made from this island spikenard and then give it to their sick slaves to drink. In most instances the slaves were soon restored to full health on account of its wonderfully revitalizing properties.

When the dried herb is given in powdered form, it helps to expel intestinal gas, cures colic, and frees the bowels from certain obstructions. The entire plant also makes "an excellent bath to take away aches and pains and heals skin ulcers" nicely.

HOLLY BERRY *(Ilex obcordata).*   As mentioned before, yaws is an endemic, infectious, tropical disease caused by the gram-negative, microaerophillic, spiral microorganism known as *Treponema pertenue*. In later stages, the skin disease is marked by lesions and patches of granulomatous papules, which may erupt again without warning. In advanced cases of yaws, there is usually destructive and deforming lesions of the skin, bones, and joints.

Negro folk healers became well acquainted with the external virtues of holly berries once they made the accidental discovery that the plant couldn't be used internally very well without producing intense discomfort and pain. A tea was made by boiling the berries, after which the skin would be frequently bathed with the strained liquid. The malady of yaws always cleared up following numerous washings.

SWEET POTATO *(Impomoea batatas).*   Lunan (2:219) wrote of the importance of this wonderful food source in the diet of slaves in this manner: "[Yams] form a considerable article of agreeable and nourishing food in the West Indies, and are generally cultivated in negro grounds only. The roots pounded are often made into a kind of pudding, called here a pone, which is baked, and, with the addition of a few ring-tailed pigeons, justly esteemed a nourishing and relishing dish. Boiled, mashed, and fermented, they make a pleasant cool drink, called mobby; and distilled afford an excellent spirit. They also make an excellent bread mixed with flour. For this purpose they are boiled till they begin to crack, or the skin peels off readily. They are then peeled and bruised while they are hot in a mortar, till not a lump remains in them."

Descourtilz (2:289) testified as to their medicinal applications. "The negroes who know how to profit from the richness, that nature is offering them at each step, cut the green stems [of young sweet potato plants] at length of two or three inches. They place those pieces into a pitched trough, designed to receive the milky sap which it expels, and congeals into a quite white resin. Others are merely content in making incisions at the foot of the plant and collecting afterwards with a spatula the resin which has congealed. By means of small incisions there transpires from all parts of the stem and the root a milky sap which congeals in the air and offers a very active purgative."

BUTTERNUT *(Juglans cinera).*   Barton described the tree's medicinal use this way: "By using the green or unripe fruit for removing the white mucalae, or white spots which often make an appearance upon the bodies of negroes, and other dark-coloured people. Also using the inner bark of the tree used as an application of a blister of cantharides to the affected parts. The spots were not only prevented from increasing, but were sensibly diminished in size, by the action of the cantharides."

LAUREL *(Kalmiella hirsuta).*   The leaves were employed by slaves and poor white folks as a cure for itch and mange in dogs. A strong decoction was applied warm to such eruptions, which usually occasioned "much smarting." Generally only one application was all that it took to effect a cure.

TULIP TREE/POPLAR *(Liriodendron tulipifera).*   The slaves of colonial Virginia gave strong decoctions of the root of this tree to horses that were troubled with worms. They also administered a syrup made from the root of this same tree to their children to promote the expulsion of intestinal parasites in general.

MAMMEE TREE *(Mammea americana).*   Lunan (1:481) and Macfadyen (1:135) both made similar observations with regard to this particular tree exudation. "A strong resinous gum [that] abounds in the bark of this tree is generally used by the negroes for extracting chigoes [chiggers] from their feet; for on being applied to the part it draws them out bag and all. Melted down with a little lime juice, and dropped into sores, it is effectual in destroying maggots at the first dressing. A bath of the bark hardens the soles of the feet like the mangrove bark."

TAPIOCA *(Manihot esculenta).*   Slaves used to boil and eat the leaves of this plant as a side dish to give them more energy and to strengthen the blood of their womenfolk (probably due to the leaves' high iron content).

WILD CUCUMBER *(Melothria guadalupensis).*   The early slaves inhabiting the Caribbean islands would collect this root, hollow it out, then fill it with rum and let it set overnight. The rum would extract all of the resin within, making it an excellent purgative where needed.

SENSITIVE PLANT *(Mimosas pudica).*   Early slaves often chewed the leaves of this plant to promote increased saliva flow that would help in the digestion of food. They would also apply hot packs of the steamed or boiled leaves to their body to relieve lumbago and nephritis. The root was regarded as a strong antidote against poison. "The negroes grind a length of four thumbs, which they [then] stir into warm wine," one account went. "This remedy produces its effect in exciting vomiting or excessive sweating" to get the poison out.

GROUND MOLE *(Modiola caroliniana).*   In the Deep South, Negro men would often employ this plant to, as they say, "bring the women right again." That meant correcting female problems such as dysmenorrhea or delayed menstruation. It was given in the form of a warm tea.

COWITCH *(Mucuna pruriens).*   This plant was a remarkable deworming agent in the early days of slavery. E. Bancroft in his *Essay on the Natural History of Guiana in South America* (London: 1769; p. 39) spoke of its medicinal applications this way: "The part used is the sebaceous hairy substance growing on the outside of the pod, which is scraped off and mixed with common syrup, or molasses, to the consistency of a thin elecruary. Of which a teaspoonful to a child of two or three years old [was then given], and double the quantity to an adult. [It] is given in the morning [while the patient] is fasting, and repeated the two succeeding mornings; after which a dose of rhubarb [root] is usually subjoined.

"This is the empirical practice of the planters, who usually once in three of four months exhibit the cowitch in this manner to their slaves in general, but especially to all their children without distinction. And in this manner I have seen it given to hundreds from one year old and upwards with the most happy success. The patients, after the second dose, usually discharge an incredible number of worms, even in the amount of more than twenty at a time, so that the stools consisted of little else than these animals. It is to be observed, that this remedy is particularly designed against long worm."

TOBACCO *(Nicotiana tabacum).*   Descourtilz (6:138) told of tobacco being used as a slave medicine in these terms: "Tobacco mixed with annatto serves for destroying vermin and chiggers who inhabit the [skin] ulcers of the negroes. They also make a decoction of the fresh or dried leaves in human urine which is then inhaled to relieve head colds. In Georgia a corncob pipe of tobacco is smoked to relieve the pain of an aching tooth. In Barbados a concentrated decoction of fresh leaves is used on ringworm and mange and also applied to the head to destroy lice."

PRICKLY PEAR *(Opuntia humifusa).*   Island slaves enjoyed eating the young leaves of this plant for nourishment. The split leaves made a good, topical emollient for relieving rheumatism and were sometimes baked and then applied hot to the skin for chronic ulcers, gout, and open wounds and sores.

AVOCADO *(Persea americana).*   Slaves in the areas of the Americas where avocado was readily available always considered it to be a great food delicacy. Long (3:308) deemed it "the favorite food with the negroes" and said it "often constitute[d] the sole support of many of the lazier [ones], who have neglected to stock their grounds with other provision[s]."

In the Out Islands of the Bahamas Negroes would boil the leaves in combination with those from *Citrus aurantifolia* (sour orange) and *Tamarindus indica* (tamarind) and then sweeten the decoction with a little sugar before taking it as a remedy against colds. In Jamaica the descendants of the early slaves still rely on the leaf decoction as a blood tonic and to relieve the distress of colds, influenza, pneumonia, and other presumably wind-related ailments. The Negroes of Panama to this day drink a decoction of the leaves and root to lower blood pressure and as a treatment for liver ailments.

Elsewhere in the Americas, slaves would chop, roast, and pulverize the avocado pit, add it to water, and drink it to stop diarrhea and dysentery. The seed powder was applied to hemorrhoids and poulticed on whitlows with good results.

ANAMU *(Petiveria alliacea).*   The slaves in the West Indies considered this to be a terrific sudorific and claimed "that vapour baths or fumigations of it will restore motion to paralyzed limbs." They also used the root as a remedy for toothache; "the negresses also employ it to produce abortion," one authority stated (but as in what form it was taken was never disclosed).

MAJOE *(Picramnia antidesma).*   Barnham (p. 96) wrote the following short treatise on this wonderful herb in 1794: "This admirable plant hath its name from Majoe, an old negro woman so called, who, with a simple decoction, did wonderful cures in the most stubborn diseases, as the yaws, and in venereal cases, when the person has been given over as incurable by physicians, because their Herculean medicines failed them, viz. preparations of mercury and antimony.

"This plant was first shown to me by a planter, who had done many excellent cures amongst his negro slaves, in old inveterate stubborn ulcers, and that by only boiling the bark and leaves, or flowers and fruit if they happen to be on the tree when wanted to make use of. [They gave] them plentifully to drink, and washing the sores with some of the decoction; then laying over them a leaf of the jack in the bush, until their sores were healed."

BITTER ASH/JAMAICAN QUASSI *(Picrasma excelsa).* W. Wright's article on the quassia simaruba tree in the *Transactions of the Royal Society of Edinburg* [2(2): 76] in 1790 mentioned this about it: "Most authors who have written on the simaruba, agree, that in fluxes it restores the lost tone of the intestines, allays the spasmodic motions, promotes the secretions by urine and perspiration, removes the lowness of spirits attending dysenteries, and disposes the patient to sleep. The gripes and tenesmus are taken off, and the stools are changed to their natural color and consistency. In a moderate dose, it occasions no disturbance or uneasiness; but in large doses it produces sickness [in the] stomach and vomiting. Negroes are less affected by it than white people."

ALLSPICE *(Pimenta dioica).* Sloane (2:76) made these few observations about this common culinary herb: "The leaves are very much made use of in baths for hydropick [dropsical or fluid-swelled] legs, etc. by the Indians, negroes and the surgeons, and may be substituted wherever bay leaves are thought useful, they resembling them in everything.

"There is no difficulty in curing or preserving of this fruit for use. The negroes and Indians climb some trees, cut down others, and pull off the twigs with the unripe green fruit, which are afterwards separated from twigs, leaves, and ripe berries, and afterwards spread on cloths exposed to the sun, from its rising to its setting for many days, whereby they become dry, rugose, and from a green, change to a brown colour, and then are fit for the market."

PEPPER ELDER *(Piper amalgo).* Lunan (2:50) quoted "as a cure for ulcers, the following observations on this plant," as given by "an anonymous writer in the *Columbian Magazine,* for the year 1798: 'Take the leaves and boil them. When boiled, beat them into a salve, which spread on one of the leaves as you would a plaster on a bit of rag. But remember first to clean well the [skin] ulcers. The water that the leaves are boiled in will answer as a bath for that purpose. Then lay on the poultice, continuing the bathing and dressing daily, and a perfect cure will be effected in a short time.'

"He also states that he knew a negro in Spanish Town [Jamaica], whose face, neck, breast, and shoulders were much ulcerated. The large orifices of the ulcers were filled up with the above described poultice. He saw her about twelve months after with the ulcers perfectly healed, and a fine child in her arms. She [told him] the cure was entirely effected by the poultice [of this plant's leaves]."

JAMAICAN BLACK PEPPER *(Piper amalago).*   One of the most amazing antivenom remedies for snakebite was mentioned by Descourtilz (3:342). To fully appreciate what he wrote, the reader may need to know something about the particular pit viper involved. The fer-de-lance is a highly poisonous snake found in tropical South America and the West Indies. It is related to the bushmaster and the rattlesnake and has heat-sensitive organs on its head for detecting its warm-blooded prey. Usually about 5 to 6 feet long, the fer-de-lance may reach a maximum length of about 9 feet. It is gray or brown with light stripes and dark diamond markings and has a yellow throat. Common throughout its habitat, it causes many human deaths; the poison is fast-acting and usually stops the beating heart and breathing lungs within minutes of being injected.

Descourtilz related the following: "I was called to treat a negro who was dying from the bite of the deadly serpent called ferdelance. I had employed all possible means, when a large negro presented himself and requested the permission to apply the remedy of their country. The malady was without hope of recovery. I saw in a few moments the venom completely neutralized by the simple application of a local remedy of Antilles black pepper [same as Jamaican black pepper]. All symptoms ceased at the third application."

The method of administration was a strong tea that had been made well in advance by boiling together the twigs, stems, and leaves for some time, straining off the liquid, and then administering the liquid *cold* to the patient three different times within a very short period.

PLANTAIN *(Plantago major).*   Several centuries ago a slave nicknamed Negro Caesar formulated through trial and error "an antidote to the effects of bites of venomous reptiles and insects" that proved so effective he later on "for [this] discovery . . . received a large reward from the Assembly in South Carolina."

MAY APPLE/WILD JALAP *(Podophyllum peltatum).*   Dr. F. P. Porcher in his *Medico Botanical Catalogue of the Plants and Ferns of St. Johns, South Carolina* (Charleston, SC: Burges and James, 1847; pp. 2; 21) made this announcement with respect to the treatment of fevers in slaves: "We have employed this plant as a substitute for jalap and the ordinary cathartics, and find that it answers every purpose, being easily prepared by the person having charge over them.

"Thirty grams of the root in substance were given or an infusion of one ounce in a pint of water, of which a wine-glassful three times a day is the dose . . . We would invite the particular attention of planters to the extensive use of [this] medicine upon the plantations. We have caused [it] to be used on one [such plantation] on which upward of a hundred negroes resided. We found that during a period of seven months, including the warm months of summer, they were used in all cases, and apparently fulfilled every indication. No detailed statement of these could be obtained, as it was administered by one of their own number. But large quantities of them were required. The soft pulp contained within the rind of the fruit has a very peculiar, musky taste, which is relished by many of the negroes."

ANTILLES FERN *(Polypodium suspensum).*   This epiphytic fern with a short-creeping and thick rhizome is brittle and covered with shiny yellow-brown hairlike scales. The fronds, which are set fairly close, are somewhat hairy and purple-brown in color. This fern grows wild on tree trunks and the stems of tree ferns in tropical forests at medium and higher altitudes.

Descourtilz (2:324) discussed some of its uses: "The application of this plant is used as a suppository in inconveniences of miscarriages. The negroes mix for this effect the very fine powder of the fern with equal parts [of] soot, equally strained, the whole melted in sufficient quantity of pine resin."

The late Mrs. Marshall, one of Jamaica's most powerful voodoo practitioners, whom I spent a week interviewing some years ago, showed me how she used the fronds: She briefly boiled them in hot water for no more than 3 minutes, set them aside to cool down to lukewarm, then strained the liquid off, added some sugar, and gave it to patients on empty stomachs to treat liver problems and syphilis. She also spoke of using the fronds in some of her "black magic" work to cast spells over others.

RED OAK *(Quercus rubra).* One source mentioned about its use: "I have myself found the bark of the tree in some service among the negroes, in several cases where a tonic astringent injection [enema] was required. [They] were using it in one of prolapsus uteri [prolapse of the uterus], where the organ became chafed and painful from exposure."

CASTOR BEAN *(Ricinus communis).* Sloane gave this commendable praise for it in passing (1:126): "'Tis good for clearing negroes skins, and for lice on the head." But it was left up to Lunan (2:13) to provide us with a much broader description of its uses by the slaves in Jamaica: "The root, decocted and drank, cures the colic and swelling of the belly and legs. So doth the leaves [likewise when] boiled with wild ginger and ground ivy, and then fermented with a little sugar or molasses, which will purge very strongly. Planters have not only cured dropsies in negroes with this drink, but also the yaws and venereal complaints, taking away the gummous nodes, and pains in the joints.

"Negroes are troubled with distemper in their legs, which they call a guinea-worm. The first appearance is a hard swelling, with much pain and inflammation. And sometime after will appear, through the flesh and skin, the head of the worm, as small as a knitting needle, which they take hold of, and draw it a little, and get it round the quilly part of a small feather. But if they draw it so hard as to break it, many ill accidents will attend the part, and sometimes gangrene ensue[s].

"Now, to ripen and forward the work, make a poultice as before directed, and lay over it one of the leaves, which will soften and bring the worm out. By turning the feather every day, drawing a little at a time, and by degrees the worm will entirely come out. It sometimes will be several yards long, and not bigger than a thread; sometimes, barely anointing the part with oil, and laying a leaf upon it, will do.

"The oil of this nut purges strongly. I knew one that would hardly give an ounce or an ounce and a half, in what they call the dry belly-ache, which would go through the patient when nothing else would. Outwardly, it is good for cold aches and pains, or cramps and contractions. Its oil will keep without being fetid or stinking, and therefore may be converted to several [other] medicines."

SUGARCANE *(Saccharum officinale).*   Lunan (2:211; 213) recorded some of its marvelous health benefits: " 'In the West Indies,' says Dr. Moseley, 'the negro children, from crude vegetable diet, are much afflicted with worms. In crop time, when the canes are ripe, these children are always sucking them. Give a negro infant a piece of sugarcane to suck, and the impoverished milk of his mother is tasteless to him. This salubrious luxury soon changes his appearance. Worms are discharged. His enlarged belly and joints [become] diminished [in size]. His emaciated limbs increase. And if canes were always ripe, he would never be diseased. I have often seen old, scabby, wasted negroes crawl from the hothouses, apparently half dead, in crop-time, and by sucking canes all day long, they would soon become strong, fat, and sleeky.

"Mr. Edwards, in his *History of the West Indies*, has very justly observed that, 'The time of crop in the sugar islands is the season of gladness and festivity to man and beast. So palatable, salutary, and nourishing, is the juice of the cane, that every individual of the animal creation, drinking freshly of it, derives health and vigor from its use. The meagre and sickly among the negroes exhibit a surprising alteration in a few weeks after the mill is set in action."

AMERICAN NIGHTSHADE *(Solanum americanum).*   The leaves of this plant were made use of by early slaves in the form of "boiled sallads," according to one source. Another put it this way: "It is daily used for food, and found by long experience to be both a pleasant and wholesome green. The negroes at the ferry make use of it every day almost [throughout] the [entire] year."

The late Mrs. Marshall, a very powerful and highly revered practitioner of the voodoo arts in Kingston, Jamaica, with whom I spent a week working and interviewing some years ago, utilized Jamaican nightshade for both medicinal and sorcery purposes.

She instructed some of her patients to make decoctions of the leaves and then bathe their leg sores with it. The fruits were made into a paste by her and applied directly to hemorrhoids and bed sores. She made a leaf infusion for asthma; the same infusion also served as an effective mouthwash to help heal canker sores on the tongue and lips. This infusion also worked well for eczema and venereal diseases.

On the witchcraft side of things, Mrs. Marshall made a juice from the leaves of this herb that she gave some of her patients to drink. A trance or profound sleep was soon induced during which time she endeavored to convince them that they possessed the power within themselves to reanimate dead bodies.

HOG-PLUM TREE (*Spondias mombin*). Long's *History of Jamaica* (2:828), published in London in 1774, reflects not only the inspiring medical knowledge of the slave folk healers, but also embraces the still deeply held prejudices of some of the white people who greatly benefitted from these remedies.

"The hog-plum tree . . . is a larger tree than any of the rest, having a large yellow plum, which hath a rankish-smell, but pleasant tart taste.

"In the year 1716, after a severe fever had left me, a violent inflammation, pain, and swelling, seized both my legs, with pitting like dropsy. I used several things [but] to no effect. A negro going through the house when I was bathing them, said, 'Master, I can cure you,' which I desired he would. And immediately he brought me the bark of this tree, with some of the leaves, and bid me bath with that.

"I then made a bath of them, which made the water as red as claret, and very rough in taste. I kept my legs immersed in the bath as long as I could, covering them with a blanket. [I] then laid myself upon the couch, and had them rubbed very well with warm napkins. I then covered them [to keep them] warm, and sweated very much [as a result]. I soon found ease and fell fast asleep.

"In five or six times repeating this method, I was perfectly recovered, and had the full strength and use of my legs as well as ever; giving God thanks for his providential care, in bestowing such virtues to mean and common plants. [But] that the knowledge of them should be made known to so vile and mean objects as negro slaves and Indians."

ARROWROOT *(Thalia genticulata).* Barnham (p. 6) recounted this unique Jamaican slave antidote for unintentional poisoning: "An accident of poison not designed, which was done by an ignorant negro slave, by stopping a jar of rum with a weed. The rum stood stopped all night, and some of the leaves fell into it. In the morning, a negro drank of it. [He] gave some to two or three more of his country[men]. In less than two hours they were all very sick with violent vomiting and trembling.

"This greatly alarmed the plantation and the master of it was sent for, letting him know that some of his negroes were poisoned, but they could not tell. He took a surgeon with him. But before he got there, two of three of them were dead, and another just expiring. The surgeon was at a stand [as] what to do. But an old negro advised Indian arrow-root, which they got immediately, and bruised it. Being a very juicy root [they were able to] press out the juice and gave it to the negro, who was seemingly a-dying.

"The first glass revived him; the second brought him to himself, so that he said he found his heart boom and desired more of it. Upon receiving the third glass, he quickly mended and in a little time recovered from his awful ordeal."

VANILLA *(Vanilla fragrans).* The slaves of the Antilles utilized the cured, aromatic pods as a natural aphrodisiac in this intriguing manner, according to Descourtilz's (8:165) account of the same: "The aroma of the vanilla is retained through rubbing the pods or more often by working them up with sugar. This is done by means of a pestle and a marble mortar. Or accomplished by simply letting them

infuse in rectified alcohol which takes possession of all its airy rudi-
ments. The negroes use it on the day of a new sexual conquest, under
the name of 'water of magnanimity' for what the men term 'getting
their natures up' [or maintaining an old-fashioned erection]."

VERVAIN *(Verbena).*   The following observations were sent to
me some years ago by Cameron Mann, a respected botanist from
Kansas City, Missouri, and are worth entering here.

"The following remedy for rheumatism was recently communicated to me by a respectable lady, who had found it quite successful
in her own case, and also with several of her friends. It was given [to]
her by an old negress who claimed many years ago to have been told
of it by an equally old Indian squaw.

"The medicine is made by boiling the root and part of the stalk of
one of the blue vervains in common vinegar for twelve hours, and
then rubbing the decoction upon the afflicted parts. Which of the
species was used I could not tell from the species shown me, as they
consisted simply of root and stalk, with, fortunately, one stalk bearing
the withered flowers. . . . The remedy certainly seems to have some
merit, whether due to the vinegar [itself] or the vervain or both. But it
undoubtedly helped several people suffering from inflammatory
rheumatism."

PRICKLY ASH *(Xanthoxylum americanum).*   This shrub or
tree can grow from 10 to 25 feet high in damp soils and tropical cli-
mates with considerable ease. As the name suggests, the branchlets
bear prickles up to a half-inch long. Small, yellowish-green flowers
growing in axillary clusters during the spring adorn the tree, before
soft, hairy leaflets and leaves appear. The fruit is a small, berrylike
capsule containing one or more shiny black seeds.

The following remarkable success with prickly ash was communicated by one Samuel Felsted to the *Royal Gazette* (an old British
newspaper formerly published in the colonial days of Jamaica, when
the island was ruled by the English), where it appeared on March 15,
1794, on p. 3.

"Mr. Crosdaile purchased two young negro wenches, in the be-

ginning of 1792. The youngest [had] at different times since been afflicted with a dry belly-ache, or colica pictonum [acute abdominal
pain due to accidental lead ingestion]. About two months ago, she
was seized with it in so dreadful a form, that our every effort to remove the spastic constriction of the bowels and procure some motions, proved quite ineffectual.

"To no purpose were emollient fomentations, anodyne or cathar-
tic clyscers, mild and drastic purges, castor oil, and ultimately blisters
to the abdomen applied. The horrid symptom of the volvulus, vomiting of the excretements, commenced and removed every ray of hope.

"In this situation she desired to have her sister with her, who,
upon seeing her deplorable condition, signified a wish of giving a
nostrum communicated to her by their Mother, and once employed to
cure herself in a similar complaint in Africa. The request I readily
complied with. In the course of two hours she returned from the
woods, with the roots and flowers (as appeared) of some plant,
pounded together in a calabash. Two spoonfuls of the expressed juice
of this she gave her sister twice, at intervals of two hours each.

"The first effect of this was a tranquil profound sleep of twelve
hours duration, during which [time] the purge and breathing gradually returned to the natural state. After this all sense of pain and every
bad symptom disappeared, and no other inconvenience did she experience, save debility and light soreness from the passing of the purgative medicines, which came away copiously during the course of the
following day. The sister was observed to boil the ingredients (after
expressing the juice) in a large quantity of water, and give it on the
following day as a common drink.

"No reward or menace could induce her to discover the plants,
until stratagem brought it to light. We induced another negro to dis-
semble a similar complaint, and prevailed with the wench to seek for
and prepare the same cure. In complying with the request, we had her
so narrowly watched, as to soon discover the secret to be the fresh
root of the [prickly ash], in its infant state. [This] was intermixed with
the saffron colored flower of the wild sage, which last, I have since
found to contribute to nothing to its virtue.

"Having procured some of the sappy and smallest roots of the young [prickly ash] trees, I expressed the juice, and began the experiment of its qualities upon myself, in teaspoon doses. From the first of these I found no other effects than an unusual flow of spirits. By continuing the dose, drowsiness, nausea, headache, etc., and at length sleep ensued. However [by the] next morning [I awoke feeling] perfectly refreshed, and had three copious easy [bowel] motions. Fearful of making any further experiments on myself, I determined my future should be on these of a different colour, and preserved some of the juice in rum and syrup. These, as well as the fresh juice, I have frequently, since that period, administered in complaints of the bowels (so frequent[ly found] among the African race and their progeny) with every wish of success.

"On the estate of Mrs. O'Brien, an old man of eighty years was lately seized with convulsive fits every hour, in every character similar to epilepsy. To him, on being sent for, I immediately gave a wineglass full of the juice preserved in rum. The fit which succeeded the first glass was unattended with strong convulsions. And the second was little else than a comatose state. After [this] a sound sleep of ten hours removed every appearance of disorder, except lassitude. This last mentioned anti-spasmodic virtue the [prickly ash] loses by being dried and powdered; its narcotic qualities being dissipated with the moisture of the plant.

"The decoction of the roots has succeeded admirably in throwing out the small pox (and has long been used by the negroes in the yaws), when such determination of the surface was thought requisite."

Valuable Contributions

The numerous botanical contributions by Black Americans have remained largely unrecognized until now. This chapter has investigated a number of important food/medicinal plants that the early slaves either brought over with them from Africa or else discovered and began using here after their arrival.

Too many of us have become accustomed to viewing black peoples primarily in an urban setting. But the data just presented reveals that their ancestors played a pioneering role in human adaption to the natural environment of the New World. We are truly indebted to them for so many natural remedies that have changed the medical landscape of healthcare ever since.

Chapter Four

THE ETHNOBOTANY OF BLACK AMERICANS

PART II: THE ART OF MAKING NATURAL PREPARATIONS

(Barbados, Dominican Republic, Haiti, Jamaica, and the Lesser Antilles)

Folk Remedies Remembered by Descendants of Former Slaves

About six summers ago, sometime in the middle of 1995, I had the good fortune to be an invited guest speaker at a national medical convention composed mostly of black physicians and practitioners. It was held in July at the Marriott Hotel closest to Disney World in Orlando, Florida. During that memorable period, I struck up friendships with a couple of elderly doctors who were nearing retirement from their profession; they had each served the black community in their particular cities for about 55 years.

One morning at a set time we met for breakfast and there discussed the subject so dear to my heart, folk medicine. Both recalled things which their own parents and grandparents had shared with them as children about their own experiences with natural cures while living on plantations as indentured servants. Their remarkable memories of such things included a number of different prescriptions for a variety of tonics, teas, and root medicines. Many of these cures were "used in an era of primitive medicine and probably represented African lore transmitted and adapted to the Southern United States," Dr. Elijah N. Williams, one of the pair, noted.

I had a little handheld microcassette recorder with me at the time and let both of them speak freely into it about the folk remedies that they could recall from their childhood days. The information in this chapter is a compilation of their recorded remarks. My other informant was Dr. Rufus K. Jones.

Slaveholders provided their slaves with doctors and medicine when needed. But usually slaves were responsible for their healthcare on a day-to-day basis. "When the slaves got sick," Dr. Jones explained, "the other slaves generally looked after them. They had white doctors, who took care of the [owners'] families, and they looked after the slaves, too. But the slaves themselves looked after each other, as a rule, whenever they took sick."

Dr. Williams chimed in next with, "When the slaves took sick or some woman gave birth to a child, herbs, salves, and home liniments were used or a midwife or old mama was the attendant. And unless there was serious sickness of some kind, most plantation owners seldom ever sent for the white doctor.

Many of the herbs used to make slave remedies are the same ones sold in health-food stores today. But slaves used herbs out of necessity and to soothe ailments associated with the hardships of their desperate lives. Constant exposure to the elements contributed to frequent respiratory and intestinal illnesses, including sore throats, colds, fevers, influenza, pneumonia, scarlet fever, dysentery, and parasites, a result of living with hogs or eating poorly cooked pork.

Often, remedies were prepared as teas. As Dr. Jones observed, "In those days, there were lots of fever cases with many folks. And they cured them and other types of sicknesses with teas made from roots, herbs, and barks that they gathered right out of the field or forest whenever needed." Dr. Williams added similar thoughts as well. "Whenever anyone came down with something serious, the old folks made hot teas from herbs taken straight from nature herself. One of them I recall was a bitter herb known as rue. This particular one was used by the slaves as an antidote to poisons and epidemic diseases such as smallpox, measles, mumps, or chickenpox."

The slaves also made plasters—dressings applied to the skin to help heal or soothe—using many of the same herbs they used to make teas with. Most often, though, they used mustard on account of the plant's strong reputation for curing respiratory disorders. A typical recipe for a mustard plaster called for one part mustard seed (powdered with the seed coats removed) to four parts whole-wheat flour and just enough liquid to make a paste, which they put in a cloth. They then applied the plaster directly over the sick person's chest to draw blood to the surface and to decrease congestion. "We both used them in our practice a long time ago," Dr. Jones admitted with a smile; his colleague chuckled a bit and nodded his head in agreement. Both of them pointed out, however, that mustard plasters shouldn't be left on the skin for very long—probably no more than 20 minutes at the most for plasters made of pure mustard powder; and perhaps 40 minutes for plasters of mustard cut with flour—since they can cause irritation and leave severe burn rashes.

Some slaveholders purchased medicine for their slaves, including castor oil, quinine, and turpentine. "Castor oil," Dr. Williams noted, "was the 'all-purpose' medicine for just about any kind of sickness that someone might come down with. Usually, one dose of that and people would get well in a hurry." Dr. Jones laughed and added: "And if any slaves still claimed to be sick, they would get an even larger dose of castor oil along with a small helping of turpentine. Those, for sure, would make someone well in an instant without much coaxing or hesitation."

Slaves routinely took these herbal tonics by the teaspoonful. Castor oil, a laxative, was commonly used by slaves, and they kept it on hand at all times, even giving it regularly to their children to purge them of impurities. They used quinine to treat nighttime muscle cramps and malaria. Pure gum turpentine (not to be confused with today's dangerous paint thinner) from fir and pine trees in the form of "spirits" was employed by them to treat toothaches, chronic bronchitis, and other ills. A small piece of cloth or wad of cotton was soaked with turpentine and then inserted into the mouth next to the aching tooth to relieve the pain. And 3 to 4 drops of turpentine were mixed in with a small pinch of sugar and placed on the tongue to slowly mix and dissolve with saliva before being swallowed to help bring up accumulated mucus from the lungs.

Also, slaves sometimes wore their herbal remedies; most often this would apply to herbs like asafetida and garlic, to help ward off disease. "I wore an asafetida bag around my neck," recalled Dr. Jones, "when I was a mere child. It was put there by my aged grandmother, who took care of me while both of my parents worked. She claimed it helped to keep away the croup, measles, diphtheria, and whooping cough." Dr. Williams joined in, "Don't forget the little muslin garlic bags they would hang around the necks of small boys and girls to keep away any type of sickness. I wore one of those myself on different occasions and absolutely *hated* it because of the stink it caused. Kids use to make fun of me in school and push and shove me around and call me 'Stinky,' which I didn't like at all."

I asked both doctors if they actually believed such nostrums worked in helping to keep young children healthier. Both of them reflected for a few moments on this question before answering it. "I think there was probably something to it," Dr. Jones said. And Dr. Williams mentioned that "I wouldn't completely rule out that some good was done by them on occasion, though I have no way of proving that."

In addition, asafetida, also called devil's dung in those days due to its very foul odor, was used as a laxative, expectorant, and digestive aid. Garlic, another equally odorous herb, enjoyed an undisputed reputation as a protector against a whole host of diseases. And when it was combined with the similarly potent asafetida, "there was a sure guarantee you wouldn't get sick," Dr. Williams pointed out.

Other sources exist elsewhere which contain numerous remedies that nineteenth-century American blacks trusted and relied upon to cure their various maladies with. In *The American Slave: A Composite Autobiography* (Westport, Conn.: Greenwood Press, 1972–1979, 41 volumes), editor George P. Rawick wrote: "Although some of the recipes seemed unpromising or bizarre, the former slaves generally placed a great deal of faith in their overall effectiveness."

Slaveholders often were suspicious of their slaves' medical remedies, but other people held these remedies in great esteem. Traditional medical practitioners recognized many of the slaves' remedies as being beneficial in some way. In the book *Roll Jordan Roll, The World the Slaves Made*, author Eugene D. Genovese reported that *Gunn's Domestic Medicine*, the medical bible of the eighteenth and nineteenth centuries, "extolled the use of herbs, and although whites, blacks, and Indians all practiced herbal medicine, the reputation of the slave medicine in the plantation districts exceeded that of the others put together."

Making Herbal Remedies the Way Slaves Did

Although some of the plants previously mentioned in this chapter may be difficult to procure, there are still enough of them readily available to use as wisdom and necessity dictate. Drs. Jones and Williams shared with me some of the ways in which they used to make a few of the simpler herbal preparations early on in their practices. The rest of the data I gathered from interviews with different elderly blacks whose parents or grandparents came from slave backgrounds and who were able to recall how things were made then.

Harvesting and Drying Herbs

The active constituents and thus the therapeutic properties themselves of botanicals can be affected by exactly when they are gathered. Medicinal plants should be harvested on a dry day, when they are at the peak of maturity and the concentration of active ingredients is highest. Dry them quickly, away from bright sunlight, to preserve the aromatic ingredients and prevent oxidation of other valuable chemicals. To ensure good air circulation, leave in a dry, airy, warm place. An airing cupboard with the door open is ideal, or a sunny room. A damp-free garden shed with a low-powered fan running can also prove just as effective. Avoid using a garage, because herbs become contaminated with gasoline fumes.

It is possible to dry herbs completely within a week's time; the longer it takes, the more likely the plant will discolor and lose its unique flavor. Keep the drying room somewhere between 70 and 90 degrees Fahrenheit. When the herbs are dry, store in clean, dry glass jars or pottery containers, with an airtight lid, out of direct sunlight. If stored when damp, the herbs will turn moldy. Label dried herbs with the variety, source, and date: most will keep for anywhere between 12 to 18 months.

Flowers.   Harvest when fully open, after the morning dew has thoroughly evaporated. Handle carefully, as they are easily damaged. Cut flower heads from the stems and dry whole on trays. Treat small flowers, such as lavender, like seeds; pick before the flowers wither completely. If the stem is large or fleshy, like mullein, remove the individual flowers and dry them separately.

When handling medicinal flowers, be sure to remove obvious dirt, grit, and insects. Spread the flowers on a paper-lined tray or newspaper to dry.

After they've dried, store them whole in a dark, airtight container. If using flowers such as marigolds, remove the dried petals and store individually, discarding the central part of the flower. But for other plants such as lavender, they may be dried on the stem in a paper bag or over a tray.

Aerial parts and leaves.   Large leaves, such as burdock, can be harvested and dried individually; smaller leaves, though, like lemon balm, are best left on the stem. Gather leaves of deciduous herbs just before flowering and evergreen herbs, such as rosemary, throughout the year. If using all the aerial parts, harvest them during their mid-flowering periods, getting a mixture of leaves, stems, flowers, and seed heads.

Tie the herbs in small bunches of about 8 to 12 stems, depending on the size, with thread or string, and hang upside down to dry. When the leaves are brittle to the touch, but not so dry that they turn to powder, rub them from the stem onto paper and discard the larger pieces. If all aerial parts are being used, crumble together. Then pour or spoon the dried herbs from the paper into an airtight storage container of some kind.

Seeds.   Harvest entire seed heads with about 5½ to 9½ inches of stalk when the seeds are almost ripe. Be sure to do this before too many have been dispersed by the wind or eaten by birds. Hang them upside down over a paper-lined tray or in a paper bag, away from direct sunlight; seeds will automatically fall off when ripe. When seed heads are hung upside down in small bunches, the seeds will usually dry within two weeks.

Roots.   Harvest most plant roots in the autumn, when the aerial tops of these herbs have wilted and before the ground becomes too hard to make digging difficult. An exception is dandelion, the roots of which should be gathered in the spring. Some roots reabsorb moisture from the air so discard them if they should become soft by chance.

Wash the roots thoroughly to remove any lingering soil and dirt. Chop larger ones into small pieces while still fresh, since they can be difficult to cut when dry. Use a clean cutting surface and a large French knife for this task. Next, spread the pieces of root on a tray lined with paper and dry for 2 to 3 hours in a cooling oven (or 4 to 6 hours for larger roots). Transfer to a warm, sunny room to complete drying.

Sap and resin.   Harvest from the tree in the autumn sometime when the sap is falling. This can be accomplished by making a deep incision in the bark or drilling a hole and collecting the sap in a tin cup tied to the tree. Sometimes a sizable bucket is required: a large amount of birch sap, for instance, can be collected overnight at certain periods of the year. Squeeze sap from latex plants such as wild lettuce or milkweed over a bowl, wearing gloves to protect your hands from their corrosive action.

When attempting to extract sap from something such an a single aloe vera leaf, carefully slice along the center off it and peel back the edges. Using the blunt edge of a paring knife, scrape the gel from the leaf and place it in a small dish.

Fruit.   Harvest berries and other fruits when they are just about but not yet fully ripe; do this before the fruit gets too soft to effectively dry. Spread on trays to dry. Turn fleshy fruit frequently to ensure even drying. Discard fruit with any signs of mold on it.

Bark. Harvest this in the fall sometime when the sap is dropping to minimize damage to the plant or tree. Never remove all the bark or a band of bark completely surrounding a tree—unless you want to sacrifice the entire botanical to herbal medicine. Never be wasteful and only take what you think you'll need; consider the plant and have regard for its welfare. Dust or wipe the bark to remove moss or insects; avoid oversoaking in water. Break bark into manageable pieces (1 to 2 inches square), spread on trays, and leave to dry.

Bulbs. Harvest after the aerial parts have wilted. Collect garlic bulbs quickly as they tend to sink downward once the leaves have wilted and are difficult to locate.

Making Herbal Remedies

The instructions given here use standard quantities of medicinal herbs. For combinations of different herbs, the total amount in any given remedy should not exceed the standard quantity. For example, an infusion for colds and influenza could contain 10 grams (⅓ ounce) each of yarrow, elderflower, and peppermint to yield the required proportion of 30 grams (about 1 ounce) of dried herb to 500 milliliters (ml) (1 pint) water.

Measuring out the appropriate amount of a particular remedy isn't rocket science and fairly easy to do. You can use any standard spoon, dropper, or measuring cup for the dosage needed. Quantities for infusions and decoctions should be divided into three equal doses.

Drop doses are usually given in amounts that equal between 5 and 10 drops depending on the age and/or condition being treated. For children and the elderly, doses should be reduced depending on age and/or bodyweight. If the individual is female and pregnant, or suffering from gastric or liver inflammation or if young children are involved, always be sure to use nonalcoholic tinctures. I've given the standard conversion equivalents for some of the metric measurements as follows:

1 ml = 20 drops
5 ml = 1 teaspoon
20 ml = 1 tablespoon
65 ml = 1 cup
130 ml = ½ cup

Infusion.   A very simple way of using herbs, an infusion is made in much the same way as tea would be. The water should be just off the boil since vigorously boiling water disperses valuable volatile oils in the steam. Use this method for flowers and the leafy parts of plants. The standard quantity should be made fresh each day and is sufficient for three doses. Drink warm or cool.

Use 30 grams (about 1 ounce) of dried herb or 75 grams (2⅔ ounces) to 500 milliliters (1 pint) of water. Standard dose should be ½ cup 2 times daily. Equipment needed for this includes: kettle, teapot, nylon sieve or strainer, teacup, and covered pitcher for storage.

Put the herb in a pot with a close-fitting lid—a teapot is ideal for this. Pour hot water over the herb. Allow it to infuse for 10 to 15 minutes, then pour through a nylon sieve or strainer into a teacup; store the rest in a pitcher in a cool place.

Decoction.   This method involves a more vigorous extraction of a plant's active ingredients than an infusion and is used for roots, barks, twigs, and some berries. Heat the herb in cold water and simmer for up to 1 hour. As with infusions, the standard quantity should be made fresh each day and is enough for 3 doses. Drink hot or cold.

Use 30 grams (about 1 ounce) of dried herb or 60 grams (slightly over 2 ounces) of fresh herb to 750 milliliters (¾ pint) water with simmering action. Standard dose should be ½ cup 3 times daily. Equipment needed includes: saucepan (preferably enamel), nylon sieve or strainer, and a covered pitcher for storage.

Place the herb in a saucepan and add cold water. Bring to a boil, then simmer for up to an hour until the volume has been reduced by one-third. Strain through a nylon sieve into a pitcher or teacup. Store in a cool place.

Tincture.   This is made by steeping the dried or fresh herb in a 25% mixture of alcohol and water. Any part of the plant can be employed for this purpose. Besides extracting the plant's active ingredients, the alcohol acts as a preservative, and tinctures will keep for up to 2 years. Tinctures should be made from individual herbs; combine prepared tinctures as required. Commercial tinctures use ethyl alcohol, but diluted spirits are suitable for home use. Slaves used corn liquor or sour mash whiskey or home brews of their own concoctions. Vodka is ideal, since it contains few additives. But don't overlook rum, which helps to disguise the flavor of less palatable herbs. If a more warming tincture is desired, go for something like brandy instead.

Use 200 grams (7 ounces) or 600 grams (21 ounces) of fresh herb to 1 liter (slightly over 1 quart) of the 25% alcohol-water mixture [e.g., dilute 75 centiliters (¾ pint) of 37.5% vodka with 37.5 milliliters (⅓ pint) of water]. Necessary equipment includes: large screw-top glass jar; jelly bag or cheesecloth; wine press; large jug or pitcher; some dark glass bottles with screw caps for airtight storage; and funnel (optional). (*Author's note:* Don't use industrial alcohol, methyl alcohol, or rubbing alcohol in tincture making. They are all *very toxic!*)

Standard dosing should be 5 milliliters 3 times daily. Tinctures should be taken diluted in water (a little honey or low-sodium V8 vegetable juice can often improve the flavor).

To make the tincture itself, first of all put the herb to be used into a large jar and cover with the vodka/water mixture. Seal the jar, store it in a cool place for 2 weeks, and shake it periodically. Next, fit cheesecloth around the rim of a wine press (securing it if necessary). Pour the mixture through it. After this, press the mixture through the wine press into a jug. The residue makes excellent compost. Finally, pour the strained liquid into some clean, dark glass bottles, using a funnel if necessary.

Now in some cases a tincture made from ethyl alcohol is unsuitable as an herbal remedy. This may be in cases of pregnancy, in gastric or liver inflammations, or when treating kids or recovering alcoholics. Adding a small amount (25 to 50 milliliters) of nearly boiling water to the tincture dose (usually 5 milliliters) in a cup and permitting it to cool effectively evaporates most of the alcohol.

Fluid extracts.   Fluid extracts are available commercially and generally not made at home as they are measured precisely to pharmaceutical grades. They are used to increase the strength of an herbal mixture when additional action is needed. Slaves never bothered making fluid extracts but contented themselves sometimes with tincture making only. Fluid extracts belong almost exclusively to the white culture.

Syrup.   This was a standard medicinal preparation in slave times and especially popular with children and elderly folks. Honey or unrefined sugar can be used to preserve infusions and decoctions. Also, syrup makes an ideal cough remedy; honey is particularly soothing. The added sweetness also disguises the flavor of more unpleasant-tasting herbs, such as rue. Syrups can also be used to flavor medicines for kids.

Use 500 milliliters (1 pint) of infusion or decoction in combination with 500 grams (17.5 ounces) honey or unrefined sugar. Standard dose is 3 times daily. Equipment needed includes: saucepan, wooden spoon, dark glass bottles with cork stoppers for storage, and a funnel (optional).

Heat 500 milliliters (1 pint) standard infusion or decoction in a saucepan. Add 500 grams (17.5 ounces) honey or unrefined sugar and stir constantly until dissolved. Permit the mixture to cool and then pour into a dark glass bottle. Seal with a cork stopper. (The cork is important, as syrups tend to ferment, and screw-capped bottles can explode.)

Infused oils.   Active plant ingredients can be extracted in oil, for external use in massage oils, creams, and ointments. Infused oils will last up to a year if kept in a cool, dark place, although smaller amounts made fresh are more potent. There are two techniques: The hot method is suitable for comfrey, chickweed, or rosemary, and the cold method for marigold and St. John's wort. If possible, repeat the process for cold infused oil using new herbs and the once-infused oil, leaving it to stand for a few more weeks before straining.

HOT INFUSION

Use 250 grams (8 ¾ ounces) of dried herb or 750 grams (about 26 ounces) of fresh herb to 500 milliliters (½ pint) of sunflower seed oil. Equipment needed includes: glass bowl and saucepan or double saucepan; wine press; jelly bag or cheesecloth; large jug or pitcher; airtight, glass storage bottles; and a funnel (optional).

Put the oil and the herb in a glass bowl over a pan of boiling water or in a double saucepan and heat gently for about 3 hours. Then pour the mixture into a jelly bag or cheesecloth fitted securely to the rim of a wine press and strain into a jug. Finally, pour the finished liquid into clean, airtight storage bottles, using a funnel if necessary.

COLD INFUSION

Use sufficient flower heads to pack a storage jar and pour over them 1 liter (slightly more than a quart) of cold-pressed oil, such as extra virgin olive oil; how much oil you use depends on the size of the jar. Equipment needed will include: jelly bag or cheesecloth or wine press; large jug or pitcher; and some airtight, glass storage bottles.

Pack a large jar tightly with the herb and cover completely with oil. Put the lid on and leave on a sunny windowsill or in a greenhouse (if one is handy) for 2 to 3 weeks. Next, pour the mixture into a jelly bag or cheesecloth, fitted snugly with string or an elastic band to the rim of a jug. Squeeze the oil through the bag. Repeat the preceding steps with new herbs and the once-infused oil; after a few weeks, strain again and store until needed.

Cream.   A cream is a mixture of water with fats or oils, which softens and blends with the skin. In the days of slavery, hog fat/lard or butter was frequently used. A good cream can be easily made with emulsifying ointment (available from most pharmacies). This is a mixture of oils and waxes that blends well with water. Homemade creams will last for several months, but the shelf life is prolonged by storing the mixture in a cool place or refrigerator or adding a few drops of benzoin tincture as a preservative.

Creams made from organic oils and fats deteriorate more quickly. Hot or cold infused oils can be thickened with beeswax, water-free lanolin, and herbal tinctures to make creams. Or the same hot or cold infused oils can be thickened with beeswax and water-free lanolin to make ointments (see next section). For a cream, though, melt 25 grams (almost an ounce) of beeswax with 25 grams of water-free lanolin, then add 100 milliliters ($\frac{1}{10}$ pint) of infused oil. Pour into clean, dark glass jars while still warm, and permit to cool.

To make the cream, melt the fats and water in a bowl over a pan of boiling water or in a double saucepan; then add the herb and heat gently for 3 hours. Next, fit a jelly bag around the rim of a wine press. Strain the mixture into a bowl. Stir constantly until cold. Finally, use a small, clean putty knife to fill the storage jars. Empty and clean baby food jars will do nicely here. Put some cream around the edge of the jar first, and then fill the middle.

Ointment.   An ointment contains only oils or fats, but no water. And unlike cream, it doesn't blend with the skin but forms a separate layer over it. Ointments are suitable where the skin is already weak or soft, or where some protection is needed from additional moisture, as in diaper rash. Slaves frequently made ointments from animals fats; hog lard was especially popular for this, but didn't keep too well and would often turn rancid in hot weather. Today petroleum jelly (Vaseline) or paraffin wax is much more suitable.

Use 500 grams ($17\frac{1}{2}$ ounces) of petroleum jelly or soft paraffin wax with 60 grams (about 2 ounces) of herbs. Equipment needed includes: glass bowl and saucepan or double saucepan; wooden spoon; jelly bag or cheesecloth; jug; and glass jars with lids.

First, melt the wax or Vaseline in a bowl over a pan of boiling water or in a double saucepan. Stir in the herbs and heat for about 2 hours or until the herbs are crisp. Then pour the mixture into a jelly bag or cheesecloth, fitted securely with string or an elastic band to the rim of a jug. Wearing rubber gloves (as the mixture is quite hot), squeeze it through the jelly bag into the jug. Finally, pour the strained mixture very quickly, while still warm and runny, into clean glass storage jars.

Powders and capsules.   Herbs can be taken as powders stirred into water or sprinkled on food. These were the usual methods employed by slaves. But today since gelatin capsules are available, they can be inserted into them and taken this way to hide the unpleasant taste of bitter herbs.

It is best to use commercially prepared powders, which are available from specialist suppliers. Grinding herbs in a domestic grinder generates heat, which can cause chemical changes in the herbs themselves. Besides this, tough roots can damage the grinder. Two-part gelatin or vegetarian capsule cases are available from specialist suppliers or some local pharmacies.

A standard size 00 capsule case holds 200 to 250 milligrams of powdered herb. Usually 2 to 3 capsules 2 to 3 times daily is the standard dosage; or ½ to1 teaspoon of herb powder in ½ glass of water 3 times a day.

To fill capsules, pour the powdered herb into a saucer. Separate the two halves of a capsule case and slide them together through the powder, scooping it into the capsule. Fit together the two halves of the capsule. Store in a dark glass jar in a cool place.

Compress.   Slaves often used a compress to accelerate wound healing or muscle injuries. A compress is simply a cloth pad soaked in a hot herbal extract and applied to the painful area. A cold compress is sometimes used for headaches. Infusions, decoctions, and tinctures diluted with water can all be used for a compress, and the pad can be soft cotton or linen, cotton ball, or surgical gauze.

Use a standard infusion or decoction or 5 to 20 milliliters of a specified tincture in 500 milliliters (½ pint) of hot water. Equipment needed will be a cloth pad and a bowl of some kind.

Soak a clean piece of soft cloth in a hot infusion or other herbal extract. Squeeze out the excess liquid. Hold the pad against the affected area. When it cools or dries, repeat the process using the hot mixture.

Poultice.   This has a similar action to that of a compress and was also popular in the indigenous folk medicine of plantation slaves. But the entire herb rather than a liquid extract is applied. Poultices are generally applied hot, but cold, fresh leaves can be just as suitable. Chop fresh herbs in a food processor for a few seconds or boil them in a little water for 3 to 5 minutes. Dried herbs can be decocted or powders mixed with a little water to make a paste.

Use adequate water to cover the affected area. Replace the poultice every 2 to 4 hours or earlier as called for. You will require a saucepan and some gauze or cotton strips for making a good poultice.

Boil the fresh herb, squeeze out any surplus liquid, and spread it on the affected area. Smooth a little oil on the skin first, to prevent the herb from sticking. Then apply gauze or cotton strips to hold the poultice carefully in place.

Steam inhalants.   These were not too common with slaves, but a few did employ them on occasion. These are ideal for conditions such as mucus, asthma, or sinusitis. Place 1 to 2 tablespoons of dried herb in a bowl and pour boiling water over it. Lean over the bowl with a towel draping over your head and the bowl. Inhale for as long as you can stand the heat or until the mixture cools. Avoid going into a cold atmosphere for at least 30 minutes.

Macerations.   Some herbs, such as valerian root, are best macerated rather than infused or decocted. Use the maceration as an infusion or decoction. Pour 500 milliliters (½ pint) of cold water over 25 grams (slightly over ¾ ounces) of dried herb, and leave the mixture in a cool place overnight; strain through a nylon sieve.

Though slaves were unacquainted with chaparral, an Indian remedy common to the American Southwest, this bitter desert herb works best against conditions such as cancer when it is macerated. Take two handfuls of dried, cut chaparral and boil them in 2 quarts of water for several minutes; then reduce the heat down to simmer and continue cooking for another 45 minutes or so. Set aside, covered with a lid, and permit to steep for 10 to 12 *hours.* Strain and drink 3 to 4 cups daily on an empty stomach for malignancies.

Skin washes.   Infusions or diluted tinctures can be used to bathe wounds, sores, skin rashes, ulcers, or other skin conditions. Soak a pad of cotton in the wash and bathe the affected area from the center outward. Slaves resorted to skin washes for all kinds of conditions. Alternatively, use a plastic atomizer to spray the herbal mixture on rashes or varicose veins.

Juices.   Slaves formerly prepared herb juices by crushing fresh plants in a mortar with a stone pestle or in a wooden bread trough using a flat, heavy stone. Today, though, herb juices can be prepared a lot easier using a food processor or a domestic juicer to pulp the plant. Squeeze the pulp through a nylon sieve or jelly bag to obtain the juice. Large quantities of the herb are needed—a 10-liter bucket (10½ quarts) of fresh herb may yield only 100 milliliter (⅒th pint) or less of juice.

Closing Thoughts

Slavery is a despicable institution which has been with mankind ever since the beginning of recorded history. It is based on a relationship of dominance and submission, whereby one person owns another and can exact from that person labor or other services. Slavery has been found among many groups of low material culture, but has also flourished in more highly developed societies, such as the Southern United States.

A revolution in the institution of slavery itself came in the fifteenth and sixteenth centuries. The explorations of the African coast by Portuguese navigators resulted in the exploitation of the African as a slave. And for almost five centuries the predations of slave raiders along the coasts of Africa were to be a lucrative and important business conducted with appalling brutality. The British, Dutch, French, Spanish, and Portuguese all engaged in this abominable trade.

African slaves were introduced to the British settlements on the Atlantic coast with the arrival of the first shipload in Virginia in 1619. The raising of staple crops—coffee, tobacco, sugar, rice, and much later, cotton—and the plantation economy made the importation of slaves from Africa particularly valuable in the Southern colonies of North America.

The slave trade then moved in a triangle. Setting out from British ports, ships would transport various goods to the western coast of Africa, where they would be exchanged for slaves. The slaves were then brought to the West Indies or to the colonies of North or South America, where they were traded for agricultural staples for the return voyage back to England. Later, New England ports were included in this last leg. From this time, on the number of slaves in the colonies dramatically increased.

The growth of humanitarian feeling during the Age of Enlightenment in the eighteenth century, the spread of the ideas of Jean-Jacques Rousseau and others, and the increase of democratic sentiment led to a growing attack on the slave trade. Believe it or not, the French Revolution had a tremendous effect not only in the spread of agitation for human rights but more directly so in the uprisings in Saint-Domingue (the modern Haiti) and the establishment of that country's eventual independence.

The movement for the abolition of slavery, despite the existence of pockets of anti-slavery sentiment, didn't have much popular support in the United States during the eighteenth and the first half of the nineteenth century. In fact, the slave trade wasn't prohibited until 20 years after the Constitution had been ratified. In the Northern states slavery eventually proved to be not only an unprofitable business venture for many, but just as equally unpopular, thanks largely to the work of the Quakers. In the South, however, things were much different. The institution of slavery came to be an integral part of the plantation system (especially after the introduction of the cotton gin in 1793).

As our nation's history has demonstrated, the issue of slavery eventually turned out to be very divisive, sectioning off the country into two great divisions—the northern states vigorously opposed to it any form and the equally passionate Deep South, which fully embraced and cherished it dearly. The Civil War was the ultimate result of this American disunion, and with the victory of the North came an end to slavery in the United States. President Abraham Lincoln's Emancipation Proclamation (issued in 1863) declared all slaves in the Southern secessionist states to be free; and it was soon followed up with the Thirteenth Amendment to the Constitution making it law and permanently guaranteeing the freedom of all formerly indentured blacks in the country.

But as history has so often proven to the case, with every great and ugly evil such as slavery also comes much good and many benefits. In this instance, it happened to have been the unique folk medicine brought by slaves from their African homelands and expanded and improved upon here in the Americas, wherever they were resettled. Our medical lore has certainly become enriched because of the many remedies that they contributed, not to mention the improvement of our nation's health overall.

As Booker Taliaferro Washington (1856–1915), a black American educationist and himself a mulatto slave in Franklin County, Virginia, one time, observed in his moderately opinionated work, *Up from Slavery* in 1901, "While slavery was certainly disgusting and unfortunate for the likes of people such as myself, yet it exercised a strange force for good in many other ways. It permitted my people to step forward and become useful citizens in a society that was often less than prepared to accept us for who we really were. It isn't so much what slavery did *to* us, but rather what we were able to do *for* the white race. We made many important contributions to society as a whole. And, as a result of our accomplishments, we were able to make America a much better place for everyone to live in, regardless of whether they were white or black."

It is then, in this cooperative spirit of mutual understanding that people of all nationalities and races today are able to enjoy many of the wonderful home remedies bequeathed to us by indentured blacks of the past. They who once were without freedom handed down to the present generation living in liberty many valuable and important pieces of folk medicine that can give release from the many ailments that continue to bind us down in the physical chains of painful suffering and emotional sorrow.

Chapter Five

EARTH MEDICINES OF THE NATIVE AMERICANS

PART I: AMERICAN INDIAN HEALING AND NUTRITION

(Flathead, Blackfoot, Okinagan, Nez Percé, and Crow Nations)

With a Soul Close to Nature

It is fitting, perhaps, to properly introduce this next section by first of all investigating the *soul* of the Native American tribes before looking at where they might have come from. No one has done a better job of this than George Wharton James in his fine book *What the White Race May Learn from the Indian* (Chicago: Forbes & Co., 1908) and Charles A. Eastman in his insightful little work *The Soul of the Indian* (Boston: Houghton Mifflin Co., 1911).

Each held similar views but declared them in his own respective way regarding the special relationship which *all* Native Americans have always held with nature in general. James said this in his chapter on the Indian and outdoor living: "The Indian is an absolute believer in the virtue of the outdoor life, not as an occasional thing, but as his regular, set, uniform habit. He *lives* out of doors; not only does his body remain in the open, but his mind, *his soul,* are ever also there."

"Virtually he sleeps out of doors, eats out of doors, works out of doors . . . except in the very cold weather. When the women make their baskets and pottery, it is always out of doors, and their best beadwork is always done in the open. The men make their bows and arrows, dress their buckskin, make their moccasins and buckskin clothes, and perform nearly all of their ceremonials *out of doors!*

"When he learns of white people shutting themselves up in houses into which the fresh, pure, free air of the plains and deserts, often laden with the healthful odors of the pines, firs, balsams of the forest, cannot come, he shakes his head at the folly. And [he] feels as one would if he saw a man slamming his door in the face of his best friend. For the outdoors of nature is and will always remain his *very best friend!*"

Eastman forthrightly declared that the typical Native American of the distant past needed no religion per se as whites, coloreds, and other races seem to require, simply because Nature herself was the only religion he ever needed. And not only did the average Native American worship nature in all of her wonderful finery, but he also lived within her presence as well.

"There were no temples or shrines among [him] save those of nature herself. Being a natural man, the Indian was intensely poetical. He would deem it sacrilege to build a house for Him who may be met face to face in the mysterious, shadowy aisles of the primeval forest, or on the sunlit bosom of virgin prairies, upon dizzy[ing] spires and pinnacles of naked rock, and yonder in the jeweled vault of the night sky! He who enrobes Himself in filmy veils of cloud, there on the rim of the visible world where our Great-Grandfather Sun kindles his evening camp-fire, He who rides upon the rigorous wind of the north, or breathes forth His spirit upon aromatic southern airs, whose war-canoe is launched upon majestic rivers and inland seas—He needs no lesser cathedral!

"The elements and majestic forces in nature, Lightning, Wind, Water, Fire, and Frost, were regarded with awe as spiritual powers, but always secondary and intermediate in character. [He] believed that the spirit pervades all creation and that every creature possesses a soul in some degree, though not necessarily a soul conscious of itself. The tree, the waterfall, the grizzly bear, each is an embodied Force, and as such an object of reverence.

"The Indian loved to come into sympathy and spiritual communion with his brothers of the animal kingdom, whose inarticulate souls had for him something of the sinless purity that we attribute to the innocent and irresponsible child. He had faith in their instincts, as in a mysterious wisdom given from above; and while he humbly accepted the supposedly voluntary sacrifice of their bodies to preserve his own, he paid homage to their spirits in prescribed prayers and offerings."

It is a fact of record that many early Native Americans did truly see in the animals of nature around them a bit of themselves, and *actually* felt that in some instances a few animals may have originally been Indians once themselves. Explorer Ross Cox, who ventured into the wild and rugged Columbia River country of what is now Oregon and Washington between 1812 and 1817, encountered a wide variety of Indian tribes, some of them hostile but others very friendly and cordial. Unlike the other mountain men and fur traders with whom he frequently associated, he himself was a man of letters, having had a good, solid education in the East during his formative years. Being thus advantaged over the others, he was able to keep detailed journals of the principal events that occurred during the greater part of this period.

His thrilling and fascinating narrative eventually made its way into print as *Adventures on the Columbia River* (New York: J. & J. Harper, 1832), an original copy of which I was able to procure from a local antiquarian bookstore a while back for $1,000. I read it through from cover to cover, not once or twice, but several times over and learned something new with each rereading.

Cox verified Eastman's prior statement that Indians of the past routinely "loved to come into . . . spiritual communion with [their] *brothers* of the animal kingdom," with this rather novel observation: "[The Flathead Indians, who then occupied the region of what is now present-day Spokane, Washington] have a curious tradition with respect to the beavers. They firmly believe that these animals are a fallen race of Indians, who, in consequence of their wickedness, vexed the Good Spirit, and were condemned by him to their present shape. But that in due time they will be restored to their humanity. They allege that the beavers have the powers of speech; and that they have heard them talk with each other, and seen them sitting in council on an offending member.

"The lovers of natural history are already well acquainted with the surprising sagacity of these wonderful animals: with their dexterity in cutting down trees, their skill in constructing their houses, and their foresight in collecting and storing provisions sufficient to last them during the winter months. But few are aware, I should imagine, of a remarkable custom among them, which, more than any other, confirms the Indians in believing them to be a fallen race.

"Towards the latter end of autumn a certain number [of beavers], varying from twenty to thirty, assemble for the purpose of building their winter habitations. They immediately commence cutting down trees; and nothing can be more wonderful than the skill and patience which they manifest in this laborious undertaking. To see them anxiously looking up, watching the leaning of the tree when the trunk is nearly severed, and, when its creaking announces its approaching fall, to observe them scampering off in all directions to avoid being crushed.

"When the tree is prostrate, they quickly strip it of its branches. After which, with their dental chisels, they divide the trunk into several pieces of equal lengths. [These] they roll to the rivulet across which they intend to erect their house. Two or three old ones generally superintend the others. And it is no unusual sight to see them beating those who exhibit any symptoms of laziness.

"Should, however, any fellow be incorrigible, and persist in refusing to work, he is driven unanimously by the whole tribe to seek shelter and provisions elsewhere. These outlaws are therefore obliged to pass a miserable winter, half-starved in a burrow on the banks of some stream, where they are easily trapped. The Indians call them "lazy beavers," and their fur is not half so valuable as that of the other busier animals, whose persevering industry and *prévoyance* secure them visions and a comfortable shelter during the severity of winter."

In our enlightened age, we know, of course, that beavers aren't humans, or vice versa (unless, of course, one subscribes to the concept of reincarnation). But to the nature-enthralled minds of primitive Flatheads and other former Native American tribes, there was a decided *human* link between themselves and members of the animal kingdom. Which idea, however superstitious, clearly showed the *tight* closeness which they had with nature in general.

Eastman was right when he wrote that "the American Indian of the past enjoyed an *intimate* association with his natural surroundings and was always on very *familiar* terms with everything living therein." Because of this there was virtually "nothing of the marvelous [which] could astonish him, [such] as that a beast should speak, or the sun stand still. The virgin birth would appear scarcely more miraculous than is the birth of every child that comes into the world, or the miracle of the loaves and fishes excite more wonder than the harvest that springs from a single ear of corn."

To the early Native American way of thinking, nature herself was the "god" whom all Indians worshipped and held a profound and sacred reverence for *all* the time, and not just when it was convenient to do so. Therefore, as we consider the different forms of "earth medicines" offered up in this chapter, let us remember that they came from a people who have always possessed a deep and abiding love for things of nature. And who have always been true environmentalists in every sense of the word, long before it became fashionable ever to be identified with such.

Native American Origins

A swirl of controversy always seems to have surrounded the true origins of the very first Native Americans. A variety of works published throughout the nineteenth century were rife with speculations as to where such a place may have been. A.J. Conant, for instance, adopted what has become pretty much the standard theory currently accepted by men and women of science. "It seems to me to be established," he wrote in his intriguing book *Foot-Prints of Vanished Races* (St. Louis: Chancy R. Barns, 1879; p. 120), "that the ancestors of the Indian tribes came to America by way of Behring's Straits."

The *London Magazine* for April 1910 contained an article by Alice Le Plongeon, the widow of Dr. Le Plongeon, who "spent many years in exploring and unearthing ruins in Yucatan." According to her, "he found the ruins of Yucatan similar to ruins found in Egypt." Furthermore, "he found that the customs of the two peoples were similar, and that the mummy of the ancient American resembles the mummy of the ancient Egyptian."

English explorers Channing Arnold and Frederick J. Tabor Frost traveled to the Yucatan and Guatemala and extensively investigated the Mayan ruins found in both places over a period of several months. Then they traveled to Cambodia and Siam (now Thailand) and spent an equal amount of time carefully evaluating the same ancient ruins in those places, with particular attention paid to those hidden deep in the hot, steamy jungles of Angkor Wat. Their record of such travels and research eventually appeared in print in England under the intriguing title *The American Egypt* (London: Hutchinson & Co., 1909), which is somewhat misleading because they assign the origins of the distant ancestors of Native Americans as coming from Cambodia instead of Egypt.

Their arguments are somewhat persuasive and worth noting here in passing. "The problem reviewed . . . is a profoundly interesting one. The ethnology of the Americas presents a problem as yet unsolved. The average ethnologist has been content to label the vast affiliated hordes and tribes of the two Americas [North and South] as Mongolian. But the American ethnological puzzle is deepened by the existence of what is known as the Mayan civilization and its many ramifications throughout Central America. Whence came these building races? And were they the forefathers of that great affiliated race of [the] American Indians?"

In drawing numerous comparisons between the old Buddhist ruins at Angkor Wat in Cambodia and the equally ancient Mayan ruins in the jungles of Guatemala, they had these singular observations to make: "A still more remarkable similarity is illustrated by a tower-like building at Yaxchilan into which is set at about the middle a huge human face. This queer edifice has probably replicas as yet undiscovered in the forests of Guatemala. If it could be shown to have a counterpart in the Malay Peninsula, that would be a connecting link between the two civilizations which would need some explaining away, would it not? Well, we have traced such a counterpart just where it ought to occur, if our theory is to hold good, *viz,* in the forests of Cambodia. At Angkor [Wat] there are several such structures built of large blocks of hewn stone. . . . It would need a bold man to say that the fact of these Cambodian towers having such a striking replica at a spot near the earliest settlements of our supposititious Oriental architects is due to coincidence.

"[At the Mayan site of Copan in Guatemala] we find the faces of the figures on the stelae are the same faces one can see today in Cambodia and Siam [now Thailand]. The dress, the ornamentation, the turban-shaped headdress (found on no other carvings but these) are all purely ancient Indo-Chinese. Couple all this with the fact that nowhere else have the counterparts of the peculiar monuments of Copan been found in Central America except at Quirigua but a few miles distant . . . and it must be admitted that there is much in our suggestion for the origins of American Indian ancestors in a remote spot like Angkor [Wat] in Cambodia or somewhere in Siam.

"In regard to the monuments themselves, a peculiar feature of the ruins of Angkor [Wat] are the gigantic heads without bodies which stand in the woods, and which have their counterparts in the heads found at Copan, one of which . . . measures about six feet in height. The carvings of Copan reached a height of elaboration and nicety of execution such as has obviously never been reached elsewhere in Central America. . . . To our mind the only way to explain the peculiar and intricate art of Copan is to assume that it was the first settlement or one of the first settlements of the first inhabitants, and where . . . we have their art in its purest and most unadulterated form. *There is sound reason, therefore, to think that most of the carvings in the ruins of Central America were done by the hands of American Indians or their ancestors.*"

I think, however, that Alexander W. Bradford provided by far one of the more sensible explanations as to Native American origins. In his book *American Antiquities* (New York: Dayton and Saxton, 1841), he drew the following conclusions at the end from all of the evidence presented in the preceding chapters of his remarkable work:

1. "Nearly all the aborigines [of the Americas] appear to be of the same descent and origin. . . . The barbarous tribes [that are now] broken [and] scattered, [are the] degraded remnants of a society originally more enlightened and cultivated."

2. ". . . Two distinct ages may be pointed out in the history of

the civilized nations [to inhabit the Western Hemisphere]. The first and most ancient, subsist[ed] for a long and indeterminate period in unbroken tranquillity, and marked towards its close by the signs of social decadence. And the second [was] distinguished by national changes, the inroads of semi-civilized tribes, the extinction of the old, and the foundation of new and more extensive empires."

3. "... The first seats of civilization [for both ages] were in Central America, whence [the] populations [were] diffused through both continents, from Cape Horn [on the extreme south] to the Arctic Ocean [in the utmost north]."

4. "... The Red [American Indian] race, under various modifications, may be traced physically to [original forebears in] Egypt ..., Mongolia, China, India, Malay[sia], Polynesia, and [even] America itself. ... The American aborigines are more or less connected with these several countries, by striking analogies in their arts, their customs and traditions, their hieroglyphical painting, their architecture and temple-building, their astronomical systems, and their superstitions, religion, and theocratical governments."

Bradford's observations seem to make the most sense in terms of the present Native American race being actually an amalgamation of genetic and cultural components from several different ancient civilizations identified with the Old World. *The Book of Mormon,* a sacred history of the different peoples who once inhabited this hemisphere (of which the American Indians are a remnant), pretty well follows the same outline given by Bradford, though in greater detail. It suggests that the so-called "mother culture" of the Americas, being archaeologically identified with the ancient Olmecs in Mesoamerica, were, in reality, a people called the Jaredites who migrated from the Tower of Babel in central Iraq around 2000 B.C. via ocean travel by barges. They were followed later in time (around 600 B.C.) by two other groups from the Middle East, one coming across the Pacific (the Nephites/Lamanites) and the other group by way of the Atlantic side (the Mulekites).

Each of these groups, in turn, had their own blend of diverse ethnicities (Aryan, Mongolian, Negro, Egyptian, Indian, Malaysian, Jewish, etc.) that accompanied them to the Americas. The continual merging and remixing of such diverse gene pools over many centuries eventually ended up producing a very unique, almost one-of-a-kind racial composite that we now identify with the Native American or American Indian.

Surgical and Medical Knowledge of the Early Native Americans

Explorer Ross Cox carefully recorded the six years which he spent among the various Indian tribes in the Pacific Northwest in his *Adventures on the Columbia River*, an extremely rare and very expensive book dealing with Western Americana. On December 24, 1813, he and some other men left the fur-trading outpost at Spokane and headed up the Flathead River some 40 miles to another trading outpost. Between Christmas and New Year's he and some of the others visited with members of the Flathead Indian nation, during which time they unfortunately witnessed the terrible torturing and ultimate deaths of several Blackfeet Indians, who had lately been taken prisoners by the former during a daring foray into enemy territory.

Cox was baffled by the names given to each tribe. "I could not discover why the *Black-feet* and *Flat-heads* received their respective designations. For the feet of the former are no more inclined to sable than any other part of the body, while the heads of the latter possess their fair proportion of rotundity."

Except for their occasional barbarity, Cox found much that was praiseworthy in the Flat-heads. "With the exception of the cruel treatment of their prisoners (which, as it is general among all savages, must not be imputed to them as a peculiar vice), the Flat-heads have fewer failings than any of the tribes I ever met with. They are honest in their dealings, brave in the field, quiet and amenable to their chiefs, fond of cleanliness, and decided enemies to falsehood of every description.

"The women are excellent wives and mothers, and their character for fidelity is so well established, that we never heard an instance of one of them proving unfaithful to her husband. They are also free from the vice of backbiting, so common among the lower tribes; and laziness is a stranger among them.

"Both sexes are comparatively very fair, and their complexions are a shade lighter than the palest new copper after being freshly rubbed. They are remarkably well made, rather slender, and never corpulent. The dress of the men consists solely of long leggings, called *mittasses* by the Canadians, which reach from the ankles to the hips, and are fastened by strings to a leathern belt round the waist. [They also] wear a shirt of dressed deer-skin, with loose hanging sleeves, which falls down to their knees. The outside seams of the leggings and shirt sleeves have fringes of leather. The women are covered by a loose robe of the same material reaching from the neck to the feet, and ornamented with fringes, beads, hawk-bells, and thimbles. The dresses of both are regularly cleaned with pipe-clay, which abounds in parts of the country, and every individual has two or three changes. They have no permanent covering for the head, but in wet or stormy weather shelter it by part of a buffalo robe, which completely answers all the purposes of a surtout (a man's long close-fitting overcoat)."

Cox quickly became an admirer of Native American medicine when one of his traveling companions, an old French Fur trapper, suffered a bite on his hand from a snarling wolf in the wild and was subsequently treated for it by an old shaman (presumably a Flat-head, though never specified).

"The wolves of this district are very large and daring. And were in great numbers in the immediate vicinity of the fort, to which they often approached closely for the purpose of carrying away the offals [animal viscera and trimmings removed during butchering]. We had a fine dog of mixed breed, whose sire was a native of Newfoundland, and whose dam was a wolf, which had been caught young, and domesticated by Mr. La Rocque, at Lac la Ronge, on the English River.

"He had many encounters with his maternal tribe, in which he was generally worsted. On observing a wolf near the fort, he darted at it with great courage. If it was a male, he fought hard; but if a female, he either allowed it to retreat harmless, or commenced fondling it. He was sometimes absent for a week or ten days; and on his return, his body and neck appeared gashed with wounds inflicted by the tusks of his male rivals in their amorous encounters in the woods. He was a noble animal, but always appeared more ready to attack a wolf than a lynx."

After providing these details, Cox then went on to mention one particularly nasty fight involving this dog and a rather large timber wolf. The hostilities became so fierce and loud at times that they drew the attention of one of the fur trappers working outside the fort at the time and not far from the scene of battle. His name was Le Clerc and, seizing a large enough stick to act as a good club, strode toward the two animals and gave the wolf a big smack on his behind with it. The injured animal let out a yelp of pain and turned quickly enough to bite his attacker on the right forearm before running away into the woods to rejoin his companions and lick his wounds.

The bite was deep and serious enough to warrant immediate medical attention; for if left unattended for very long, it could lead to high fever, delirium, and major infection. An old, wizened shaman of many years, who just happened to be in the fort at the time this incident happened, came forward and volunteered in his native tongue to treat the problem. All of the white men present agreed to this, knowing that the surgical and medical knowledge of the local Indians far surpassed their own and, in many instances, was even far superior.

The first thing the old medicine man did was to make several incisions around the site of the bite itself, to let the blood flow freely for several minutes. After which the area was roughly washed with half a cup of rum. The shaman went some distance into the woods and returned a few minutes later carrying some dug roots of barberry or wild Oregon grape (*Berberis aquifolium*). He brushed away most of the dirt with his hands and then proceeded to cut up the roots into small pieces and place them in the bottom of an iron pot. He took a large wooden mallet and proceeded to pound the roots until they were thoroughly mashed.

After this, he scooped them up into one hand and slowly let some of his own spittle drop from his mouth onto the mashed pulp, which he stirred in with the forefinger of his other hand. The purpose of the saliva was probably to help the mixture stick better to the skin. The entire wet mass was then placed upon the injured site and bound in place with a strip of cloth. The old Indian also gave instructions for the remaining root pulp to be boiled with some water and given to the French trapper to drink. Cox reported that by the following day their companion was doing quite well and had not experienced any of the symptoms which typically follow such an unattended wound from a wild animal.

"The Flat-heads are a healthy tribe, and subject to few diseases," Cox wrote of their benefactors and friends. "Common fractures, caused by an occasional pitch off a horse, or a fall down a declivity in the ardour of hunting, are cured by tight bandages and pieces of wood like staves placed longitudinally around the part, to which they are secured by leathern thongs. For contusions they generally bleed, either in the temples, arms, wrists, or ankles, with pieces of sharp flint, or heads of arrows. They however preferred being bled with the lancet, and frequently brought us patients, who were much pleased with that mode of operation of the white man.

"Very little snow fell after Christmas. But the cold was intense, with a clear atmosphere. I experienced some acute rheumatic attacks in the shoulders and knees, from which I suffered much annoyance. An old Indian proposed to relieve me, provided I consented to follow the mode of cure practiced by him in similar cases on the young warriors of the tribe. On inquiring the method he intended to pursue, he replied that it merely consisted in getting up early every morning for some weeks, and plunging into the river, and to leave the rest to him.

"This was a most chilling proposition, for the river was firmly frozen, and an opening to be made in the ice preparatory to each immersion. I asked him, 'Would it not answer equally well to have the water brought to my bedroom?' But he shook his head, and replied he was surprised that a young white chief who ought to be wise, should ask such a foolish question. On reflecting, however, that rheumatism was a stranger among Indians, while numbers of our people were martyrs to it, and, above all, that I was upwards of three thousand miles from any professional assistance, I determined to adopt the disagreeable expedient, and commenced operations the following morning.

"The Indian first broke a hole in the ice sufficiently large to admit us both, upon which he made a signal that all was ready. Enveloped in a large buffalo robe, I proceeded to the spot, and throwing off my covering, we both jumped into the frigid orifice together. He immediately commenced rubbing my shoulders, back, and loins. My hair in the meantime became ornamented with icicles. And while the lower joints were undergoing their friction, my face, neck, and shoulders were encased in a thin covering of ice.

"On getting released I rolled a blanket about me, and ran back to the bedroom, in which I had previously ordered a good fire. In a few minutes I experienced a warm glow all over my body. Chilling and disagreeable as these matinal ablutions were, yet, as I found them so beneficial, I continued them for twenty-five days, at the expiration of which my physician was pleased to say that no more was necessary, and that I had done my duty like a wise man. *I was never after in my life troubled with a rheumatic pain!*

"One of our old Canadians, who had been labouring many years under a chronic rheumatism, asked the Indian if he could cure him in the same manner. The latter replied it was impossible, but that he would try another process. He accordingly constructed the skeleton of a hut about four and a half feet high and three broad, in a shape like a beehive, which he covered with deer-skins. He then heated some stones in an adjoining fire, and having placed the patient inside in a state of nudity, the hot stones were thrown in, and water poured on them. The entrance was then quickly closed, and the man kept in for some time until he begged to be released, alleging that he was nearly suffocated. On coming out he was in a state of profuse perspiration. The Indian ordered him to be immediately enveloped in blankets and conveyed to bed. This operation was repeated several times, and although it did not effect a radical cure, the violence of the pains was so far abated as to permit the patient to follow his ordinary business, and to enjoy his sleep in comparative ease."

These Native Americans were not without their own unique version of religion, as Cox amplified in his book. "The Flat-heads believe in the existence of a good and evil spirit, and consequently in a future state of rewards and punishments. They hold, that after death the good Indian goes to a country in which there will be perpetual summer. [There] he will meet his wife and children. [There] the rivers will abound with fish, and the plains with the much-loved buffalo. And [there] he will spend his time in hunting and fishing, free from the terrors of war, or the apprehensions of cold or famine.

"The bad man, they believe, will go to a place covered with eternal snow. [There] he will always be shivering with cold, and will see fires at a distance which he cannot enjoy. [There he will also find] water which he cannot procure to quench his thirst, and buffalo and deer which he cannot kill to appease his hunger. An impenetrable wood, full of wolves, panthers, and serpents, separates these 'shrinking slaves of winter' from their more fortunate brethren in the 'meadows of ease.' Their punishment is not however eternal, and according to the different shades of their crimes they are sooner or later emancipated if they repent of their bad behavior, and [then] permitted to join their friends in the Elysian fields.

"Their code of morality, although short, is comprehensive. They say that honesty, bravery, love of truth, attention to parents, obedience to their chiefs, and affection for their wives and children, are the principal virtues which entitle them to the place of happiness, while the opposite vices condemn them to that of misery."

Later in his spell-binding book, Cox introduced readers to some of the native remedies that then belonged to the Okinagan Indians who occupied pretty much all of the land that now forms Okanogan County in the upper part of Washington State. "On the 16th of April we took our departure for the interior. Our party consisted of sixty-eight men, including officers. . . . We arrived at Oakinagan on the 30th [of April 1816].

". . . I [had been] selected as commandant of [this] place. . . . A sufficient number of men [came] with me for all purposes of hunting, trading, and defence. . . . I had a long summer before me. It is the most idle season of the year. And it was intended to rebuild and fortify Oakinagan [fort] during the vacation. I lost no time in setting the men to work. . . . The point of land upon which the fort is [being re-built] is formed by the junction of the Oakinagan River with the Columbia [River]."

In an atlas this location of which Cox spoke can be located on a political map of Washington State: It is just a couple of miles to the east of the tiny town of Brewster and forms a portion of the natural borders of Okanogan and Douglas Counties. "The point is about three miles in length and two in breadth," he wrote. "At the upper end is a chain of hills, round the base of which runs a rocky pathway leading to the upper part of the river. Rattlesnakes abound beyond these hills, and on the opposite sides of the Oakinagan and Columbia rivers. They are also found on both sides of the Columbia, below its junction with the former stream. But it is a curious fact, that on the point itself, that is, from the rocks to the confluence of the two rivers, a rat-tlesnake has never yet been seen.

"Immense quantities of sarsaparilla grow on Oakinagan Point, which at times proved very beneficial to some of our [men]." This isn't to be confused with the true sarsaparilla belonging to the *Smilax* species; rather it was the plant *Aralia nudicaulis,* which was also called sarsaparilla in the early times of the mountain men and fur trappers.

Cox reported that this wild sarsaparilla was widely employed by the Indians of the region for a variety of purposes. "The bark of the roots . . . is of a bitterish flavour, but aromatic. It is deservedly es-teemed for its medicinal virtues, being a gentle sudorific [an agent that increases sweating], and very powerful in attenuating the blood when impeded by gross humours [excess bile and phlegm]. . . . The Indians [around here] subsist upon them for a long time, in their war and hunting excursions. . . . The root is used in medicine [as a decoc-tion] for wounds, and its virtues are well known. . . . The [Indian] women cut up the roots, tie the pieces with a strip of leather, and keep them in their lodges until needed. The root is [sometimes] made into a decoction and used to bathe eyes made sore from the wind and sun. . . . I have seen the root pounded to make a poultice for burns and sores with good effect. It is mixed with the inner bark of the prickly ash tree and barberry [wild Oregon grape] to give strength to them who are weak in body. The pounded root is poulticed on swellings and infections with good effect."

Cox continued his thrilling narrative with more, shall I say, "tasty" information about the many snakes to be found in the region. "Numbers of black snakes are found on the point, but they are perfectly harmless. We caught some of them in the rooms, and a few have been found at times quietly coiled up in the men's beds; I found one inside my moccasin one morning. The rattlesnakes were very numerous about the place where the men were cutting the timber. I have seen some of our Canadians eat them repeatedly! The flesh is very white, and they assured me, had a most delicious taste. Their manner of dressing them is simple. They at first skin the snake in the same manner as we do eels, after which they run through the body a small stick, one of which is planted in the ground, leaning towards the fire. By turning this *brochet* occasionally, the snake is shortly roasted. Great caution however is required in killing a snake for eating. For if the first blow fails, or only partially stuns him, he instantly bites himself in different parts of the body, which thereby becomes poisoned, and would prove fatal to any person who should partake of it. The best method is to wait until he begins to uncoil and stretches out the body, preparatory to a spring; when, if a steady aim be taken with a stick about six feet long, it seldom fails to kill with the first blow.

"The climate of Oakinagan is highly salubrious. We have for weeks together observed the blue expanse of heaven unobscured by a single cloud. Rain, too, is very uncommon; but heavy dews fall during the night."

In this place, Cox and his men encountered the Okinagan tribe, which he described as being "quiet and friendly." In fact, he felt that the area which the Indians had selected to settle in was "a spot preeminently calculated for the site of a town, when civilization (which is at present so rapidly migrating towards the westward) crosses the Rocky Mountains and reaches the Columbia [River basin]."

He took particular note of these Indians and spoke favorably of their virtues, as well as mentioning great shrewdness when it came to trading with the white man.

"The natives of Oakinagan are an honest, quiet tribe," Cox observed. They do not muster more than two hundred warriors. . . . Their principal occupations consist in catching and curing salmon, and occasionally hunting for deer and beaver, neither of which abounds on their lands. Acts of dishonesty are of rare occurrence among either men or women; and breaches of chastity among the latter are equally infrequent.

"Their manner of trading [with the white man] resembles that of most other tribes. A party arrives at the fort loaded with the product of their hunt, which they throw down, and round which they squat themselves in a circle. The trader lights the calumet of peace, and directing his face first to the east, and so to the other cardinal points [of the compass], gives at each a solemn puff. These are followed by a few short quick whiffs, and then he hands the calumet to the chief of the party, who repeats the same ceremony. The chief passes it to the man on his right, who only gives a few whiffs, and so on through the whole party until the pipe is smoked out. The trader then presents them with a quantity of tobacco to smoke *ad libitum,* which they generally finish before commencing their barter, being, as they say themselves, 'A long time very hungry for a smoke.'

"When the smoking terminates, each man divides his skins into different lots. For one, he wants a gun; for another, ammunition; for a third, a copper kettle, an axe, a blanket, a tomahawk, a knife, ornaments for his wife, etc., according to the quantity of skins he has to barter.

"The trading business being over, another general smoking-match takes place; after which they retire to their village or encampment. They are shrewd, hard dealers, and not a whit inferior to any native of Yorkshire, Scotland, or Connaught, in driving a bargain."

What is to follow next, while exceptionally interesting if not somewhat strange pertaining to Indian healing skills of the time, may not be for everyone's reading tastes. This is especially applicable to animal lovers, or those easily disturbed by what they may perceive to be acts of extreme animal cruelty (which the people then viewed in a much different light than we do now). These particular medical narratives take up the next few pages, and while certainly instructive in one sense, may also prove revolting to some individuals on the other hand. Therefore, "discretion being the better part of valor," proceed reading the rest of Cox's excerpts at your risk and cautious judgment!

"The Oakinagan mode of curing some of our diseases would probably startle many of the faculty. The following case in particular passed under my own observation:

"One of the proprietors had, in the year 1814, taken as a wife a young and beautiful wife, whose father had been one of the early partners, and whose mother was a half breed (her grandmother having been a native of the Cree tribe). So that, although not a pure white, she was fairer than many who are so called in Europe. He proceeded with her to Fort George; but the change of climate, from the dry and healthy plains of Forts des Praires to the gloomy forests and incessant rains on the north-west coast, was too much for her delicate frame, and she fell into a deep consumption. As a last resort, her husband determined to send her to Oakinagan to try the change of air, and requested me to procure her accommodation at that place for the summer. This I easily managed. She was accompanied by a younger sister, and an old female attendant.

"For some days after her arrival we were in hourly expectation of her death. Her legs and feet were much swollen, and so hard that the greatest pressure created no sensation. Her hair had fallen off in such quantities as nearly to cause baldness. A sable shade surrounded her deeply sunk eyes. She was in fact little more than a skeleton, with scarcely any symptoms of vitality, and her whole appearance betokened approaching dissolution.

"Such was the state of the unfortunate patient, when an old Indian, who had for some days observed her sitting in the porch-door, where she was brought supported on pillows to enjoy the fresh air, called me aside, and told me he had no doubt of being able to cure her provided I would agree to his plan. But [then he] added, that he would not give any explanation of the means he intended to use, for fear we might laugh at him, unless we consented to adopt them. We accordingly held a consultation; the result of which was, that the Indian should be allowed to follow his own method. It could not make her worse, and there was a strong possibility of success, knowing that these people are highly skilled in the healing arts.

"Having acquainted him with her acquiescence, he immediately commenced operations by seizing an ill-looking, snarling, cur dog, which he half strangled; after which he deliberately cut its throat. He then ripped open the belly, and placed the legs and feet of the patient inside, surrounded by the warm intestines, in which position he kept them until the carcass became cold. He then took them out and bandaged them with warm flannel, which he said was 'very good.'

"The following day another dog lost its life, and a similar operation was performed. This was continued for some time, until every ill-disposed cur in the village had disappeared by the throat-cutting knife of our dog-destroying doctor, and we were obliged to purchase some of a superior breed. While she was undergoing this process, she took, in addition, a small quantity of red [slippery] elm [*Ulmus fulva*] inner bark daily in a glass of port wine. In the meantime the swelling gradually decreased, the fingers lost their corpse-like nakedness, the hectic flushes became rarer, and 'that most pure spirit of sense,' the eye, gave evident tokens of returning animation.

"When her strength permitted, she was placed on the carriage of a brass field-piece, supported by bolsters, and drawn occasionally a mile or two about the prairie. The Indian continued at intervals to repeat this strange application, until the swelling had entirely disappeared, and enabled her once more to make use of her limbs.

"Two-and-thirty dogs lost their lives in bringing about this extraordinary recovery, and among them might truly be numbered

> Mongrel, puppy, whelp, and hound,
> And curs of low degree.

"She gradually regained possession of her appetite. And when her husband arrived in the autumn from Fort George, for the purpose of crossing the mountains, she was strong enough to accompany him. The following summer, on my journey across the continent, I met them at Lac la Pluie. She was in the full enjoyment of health, and 'in the way which ladies wish to be, who love their lords.'

"Before I quit this subject I may be permitted to mention another remarkable cure by means nearly similar, which occurred at Fort

George. One of the proprietors, who had been stationed there for two years, had, like his countryman Burns, an unconquerable '*penchant à l'adorable moité du genre humain.*' And among the flat-headed beauties of the coast, where chastity is not classed as the first of virtues, he had unfortunately too many opportunities of indulging his passion.

"His excesses greatly impaired his health, and obliged him to have recourse to the most powerful medicine of the *materia medica.* His constitution was naturally weak, and the last attack was of so serious a nature, as to deprive him for many days of the powers of articulation. The contents of the medicine chest were tried in vain, and all hopes of his recovery had been abandoned, when a Clatsop Indian undertook to cure him.

"Mr. M—— consented, and a poor horse, having been selected as a sacrifice, was shot. The Indian then made an opening in the paunch sufficiently wide merely to admit the attenuated body of the patient, who was plunged in a state of nudity into the foaming mass of entrails up to the chin. The orifice was tucked tightly about his neck to prevent the escape of steam, and he was kept in that situation until the body of the animal had lost its warmth. He was then conveyed to bed, and enveloped in well-heated blankets.

"The following day he felt considerably better. In a few days afterwards another horse suffered. He underwent a second operation, which was attended by similar results. From thence he slowly regained his strength. And by adhering to a strict regimen, [he] was finally restored to his ordinary health. Horses are scarce at Fort George, were it not for which circumstance, Mr. M—— assured me he would have killed two or three more for the beneficial effects they produced on his constitution. His late illness, however, was so dangerous, and his recovery so unexpected, that it checked for the future his amatory propensities."

The preceding incidents involving slaughtered dogs and horses for the purpose of restoring vitality depended largely upon the internal heat generated by these sacrificed animals. Today such drastic measures wouldn't be as necessary, provided that *warm* baths (full, half, sitz, foot and hand) consisting of herbal solutions or Epsom salts could be used in their place. Such medicinal baths have been extremely popular in Europe for a number of centuries and have proved themselves very efficacious in the treatment of many different illnesses, as well as restoring a certain amount of vitality to bodies seemingly on the verge of death. Plain warm water won't work as well; there must be something else in it to manifest "drawing power" as the butchered animals did.

Absarog-Issawua (From the Land of the Crow Indians)

Legend has it that the remote ancestors of the Crow Indians once lived in a land of forests and many lakes; it is believed by most tribal members that this ancestral home was near what is now Lake Winnipeg, Canada. Around A.D. 1550, their ancestors migrated in a southwestward direction across the Great Plains. Their medicine men sought the help of the Great Spirit for guidance in their long trek. They were instructed by Him to move westward until they came to occupy the vast stretch of land lying between the Black Hills of South Dakota and the Rocky Mountains of Montana and Wyoming, and between the North Platte River in Wyoming and the Milk River in northern Montana. It was in this huge territory that they freely roamed, hunting bison and waging war against their enemies.

The Crow, although always smaller in numbers than other Indian tribes of this region, were one of the strongest military powers on the Great Plains. In fact, being one of the smallest of the Plains tribes may have been one of the circumstances that led them to become so militaristic. They became expert horsemen and generally owned more horses than did most other Indians of the Plains. Communal hunts were frequent and carefully planned well in advance; they helped to provide the necessary food, clothing, and shelter on which these people depended for so long.

But with the ever-increasing push of white people westward, the Crow were one of the very first tribes to realize early on that it was better to make "peace" (however temporary) with your enemy than to resist him; as a result, Crow chiefs signed the first Treaty of Fort Laramie in 1851 with U.S. government officials, promising never to make war on the white man again—a promise which they kept, by the way. In return for their loyalty, they received 38.5 million acres of reservation land, almost half the present state of Montana. But over the last century, the Crows managed to lose 36.3 million of those acres to unscrupulous ranchers, mining companies, and government agencies.

Today, some 6,700 members of the tribe live on 2.2 million acres of mountains and high rolling prairies in southeastern Montana in what is referred to as the Crow Agency. The people whom American explorers Lewis and Clark once described as being "the finest horsemen in the whole world" live in rickety government-built housing and exist on welfare and food stamps, for the most part. Unemployment hovers around 65 percent most of the time; the average annual income is about $3,000.

Although the Crow, who call themselves *Absaroga* or "Bird People," from which comes their official tribal name, face a bleak life in general, their reservation sits on $26.7 billion worth of untapped coal, oil, gas, and other mineral assets. Strapped for cash, Crows are quick to lease reservation land to whites for grazing, haying, logging, and mining.

Over two decades ago the Crows finally awakened to the fact that education might help them in dealing with cunning whites, but the nearest college was then in Billings, a 120-mile round trip from the Crow Agency. It might as well have been across the world. The Crows have an almost mystical bond to family, community, and their land. The few who were able to attend college were taught white values by white professors in a white world filled with greed, vanity, and self-importance. The Crows faced a dilemma: how to get the education necessary to cope in the white man's world, yet retain their own personal dignity and tribal heritage.

In 1978 the Crow Nation applied for a federal grant to start a two-year college that would educate Crows in their ancient culture and in survival skills for the modern world. (Until the Tribally Controlled Community College Act of 1978, the few Indian colleges that existed were run either by the government or by religious groups.) Over two decades later, Little Big Horn College, one of 25 Indian-run colleges in the country, offers associate degrees in nine different fields of study. Fall, winter, spring, and summer quarters usually average 150 to 225 students per quarter.

Many of the college's 127 courses are taught in Crow (the first language for 85 percent of the tribe). In addition to such traditional college staples as math, economics, statistics, sociology, psychology, and journalism, students are encouraged to take practical courses—home economics, first aid, parenting, carpentry, and welding. Some of the most popular offerings, though, are in the Crow Studies Department: Crow Literature, Crow Dance, History of the Crow Chiefs, Indian Identity and Awareness, and until only very recently, Traditional Foods and Medicines.

One of the tribal members responsible for pioneering this work back in the late 1970s and 1980s was Joy Yellowtail Toineeta. I had the good pleasure and privilege of spending nearly two weeks interviewing and working with her in the midsummer of 1975. Once she was able to get by her early suspicions of why a white anthropologist like myself was so interested in the native diet and folk medicine of her people, and became fully convinced that my purposes were genuine and noble, she was very forthcoming and helpful after that. What follows, therefore, was valuable data carefully gleaned from that precious visit that is now appearing for the very first time in print that I know of. My kind benefactor passed away some years ago, but her work and legacy live on in a book such as this.

I remember her telling me, "Our people believe in sharing things with each other, because it is the right way to live and do things. You are non-Indian and not even Crow. I am doing this, not for you or even for myself, but for my people and other non-Indians in your world. I believe that the Great Spirit intended us to help others, even if they don't necessarily belong to your particular tribe. Not all Crow feel or think as I do. Your experience with that other tribal healer, who told you to 'go to hell' and drove you off his property, is still the thinking of many healers here unfortunately. But my grandmother told me when I was a young woman that in order to be always found in the favor of the Great Spirit, one had to be kindly disposed and willing to assist where it seemed practical to do so.

"You could not pay me for the things I have been sharing with you and showing you so far. No amount of money could ever persuade me to do that. I freely received these things from my grandmother, who was gifted with the powers of healing. She received some of her knowledge about native plants from her own mother; but the healing power itself came to her through a vision, as is the case with other healers.

"She clung tenaciously to the old religious beliefs of our people, which are fast disappearing. They were once very much a part of daily Crow life. To obtain her vision quest, she went through a period of personal preparation involving fasting and purification. She made sure this was done during a period in which she wasn't menstruating; our people use to believe that a healer couldn't obtain a healing vision if the person had engaged in sex or menstruated beforehand.

"My grandmother told me that in 1904 the United States government decreed that the healing of the sick and injured by 'medicine people' like her was to be considered a criminal offense. But the Crow healers still managed to continue their practice, but only in secret. And while you are correct in stating that most tribal healers have been men, there have been a few women included in this sacred profession, my grandmother being one of them."

Nutritive Foods for Regaining Wellness

One of the food remedies which was constantly employed by her grandmother for the recuperation from serious illness in old and young alike was called *ganuge* or *conutchee,* it being a delicious and reviving gruel made from hickory nuts. Joy Yellowtail gave the instructions for making it as follows: "Pulverize whole hickory nuts until they can be processed together by hand to form a ball. To make the medicine gruel, cook some hominy grits in a heavy cast iron kettle over an open fire until done. Then take one or two of the hickory balls and cover with boiling water in another kettle. Stir constantly. When the nuts disintegrate in the hot water, some of the hulls will float to the top. Sieve this gruel to remove the hulls. Then add the strained hickory gruel to the hominy.

"If this makes into a thick soup, it may be served with whole wheat bread or wheat dumplings. If it is made into a thin soup for the severely ill who can't digest heavier food too well, then administer it in the form of a warm drink every 3 hours. As the thin soup is poured off, more water can be added. This last of this mixture is not edible as there may be bits of hull [in it]."

Ms. Toineeta's grandmother relied a great deal on vegetables, mostly sun-dried, presoaked, and then cooked to help sick people regain their strength. She said that her grandmother felt that "nutritious herbs" (as she called vegetables) were just as important in the healing process as were more traditional medicinals such as bear root. The data below and on the next several pages comes just as Joy Yellowtail (the name by which she went most often) wrote it out for me almost three decades ago in her home on the Crow Agency in southwestern Montana.

"All of the vegetables that the Crow Indians used were gathered early in the spring, prepared and dried in the sun to preserve for winter. My grandmother was busily engaged in this occupation as part of her healing responsibilities.

"The wild turnip which the Crow called Ee-hay and the botanist named *Psoralea argophylla,* is a root vegetable that grows best in sandy soil on hillsides. The size of the root varies from slender pencil size to the proportion of a large cultivated Oxheart carrot. The skin is smooth when quite small but becomes tough and woody when it reaches maturity. The root is dug early in June after the spring rains when the plant is in bloom; this is when the root reaches its peak in flavor. It is firm and peels easily. It is sweet to the taste and retains its natural flavors. The name 'wild turnip' is misleading because it does not resemble the turnip in texture, flavor, or in any other way.

"To use the root, the skin is peeled off and the white, firm, starchy root is sliced off to the core. The slices are then dried in this form or pounded and mashed to a coarse meal, then spread out in the sun to dry. A stone mallet and a rawhide vessel, shaped like a large dish pan, served as a good chopper for my grandmother in the old days. Today, whenever I use some of this to help someone get well again, I put it through the food chopper. The coarse meal is then sacked in cellophane freezer bags and stored in the deep freeze, or sun dried and stored in airtight containers.

"The wild turnip can be eaten fresh. It is quite dry and starchy, but filling. When carbohydrate foods are called for in certain cases of sickness, this is one of the best to use. Its nutritive powers bring on recuperation and are amazing.

"To prepare this or any vegetables, it is more nutritious as well as flavorsome, to cook them in a stock prepared from cracked marrow bones. Nothing was wasted from any game that Crow hunters brought home in the old days. My grandmother claimed (and I believe her) that marrow bones contain more healing nutrition in them than just about anything else around.

"She saved the bones from which she removed the meat to make jerky. While the sliced meat—buffalo, venison, rabbit—was drying in the sun, she cracked the marrow bones, boiled them, and removed the fat to use later in pemmican, or to add to her vegetables as a cook adds butter to her carefully steamed vegetables today.

"This stock is the liquid in which the vegetables are cooked until done. This is thickened with the white shavings from the second layer of skin that the tanner saved from dressing a hide. This cooks into a gelatinous substance. The modern day cook uses flour or cornstarch for thickening.

"Not many Crow Indians cook cracked marrow bones [anymore] for the stock to cook native root vegetables and fruit. Water from the tap or well is used instead. Soaking the dried vegetables enhances the flavor and shortens the cooking time. My grandmother persisted in using the old ways and taught me that they were always the best to use; she wasn't much impressed with the way modern cooks do things now. I still use cracked marrow bones to prepare certain root vegetables for feeding the sick when I'm called upon to treat them."

Joy's method of preparing wild turnip is based on the same recipe handed down from her long since deceased grandmother. "Soak 2 cups of ground turnip meal [see preceding recipe] in 2 cups or 3 cups of warm water until the particles are soft and swollen. Let simmer over medium heat until the vegetable is tender, about 1 hour. Mix cup of whole-wheat flour with enough water to form a smooth paste. Add this to the cooked turnip, stir vigorously to prevent lumping, cover, and let boil 5 minutes. Add 2 tablespoonsful of bone marrow fat and remove from fire. This is best sweetened with a little honey. Serve to your sick patient warm."

Wild parsley or black root was a food favorite with sick children and the frail elderly, as it was a food they could easily digest and found quite tasty when properly prepared. "Marshaspita is what we call it in the Crow language," Joy spoke into my tape recorder. "It means 'that which has black root' (*Musineon divaricatum*). This plant has a fleshy root. It is dug when it is in bloom. It grows in open meadows, where sweet grass grows that the deer, elk, and even bears like to graze on. It is starchy and has a pleasant and sweet flavor eaten fresh. This plant can be cooked like the other roots. The almost black cuticle or skin peels off easily, but it can be eaten too. The roots are washed clean and boiled, and mashed when cooked. Then thicken a little and add a small amount of cracked bone marrow."

Rose hips, or *mitch-gub-ay* as they're known by the Crow name, have always been a real favorite for tribal healers. "The literal translation once was 'dog's nose,'" Joy informed me with a hearty laugh. "But due to changes in our language over the many years, the true meaning has been lost. The botanical name is *Rosa nutkana*. The fruit is gathered and utilized by Crows for food after the first frost and during wintertime. The hips are stewed in stock or water, mashed when cooked with a potato masher, and thickened with wheat flour paste; a tablespoonful of animal fat or bone marrow is added, with a little honey, to improve flavor.

"As you probably know yourself, Dr. John, it is always difficult giving young children who are sick any type of food or medicine that doesn't taste 'right' to them. It is no different in our world than in yours—Crow children can be just as fussy about having to take something they think is bad tasting or awful smelling, no matter how good it may be for them. My grandmother made this next food remedy up for children with fever, coughs, or colds. It is made out of rose hips and is good for them.

"Four cups of berries are needed for this Rose Hips Concentrate; they are mashed between two thicknesses of clean canvas about one-half yard square. Use a hammer or hatchet to mash the berries. Wash the hammer or hatchet. A food chopper may be used. Add to the mashed berries 2 cups of kidney fat that has been broken up in small pieces. Mash the two together until mixed well, then add 1½ cups of wild honey and mix well with the hands. The honey will make the mixture sticky. More honey may be added to suit children's tastes. The concentrate is now ready to form into oblong balls. Put them in a pan and store in the refrigerator until 'set' and until the balls do not stick to the hands.

"To eat these balls, use a clean stick about 2 feet long or a long picnic fork. Spear the balls lengthwise and roast closely over the open fire or over a bed of hot coals until the surface is brown and bubbly. It will be very hot so let it cool until it is comfortable for a child to lick. The seeds should be spit out as this is done. Then return over the fire or hot coals to roast this rose hip ball. The child should lick it again and then continue roasting until he is finished with it. This has combined flavors of delicious apples and strawberries. The modern food chopper will do a good job of grinding and mashing the berries and suet together. Among the Crow these are known as 'Medicine Marshmallows.' "

Pumpkin and squash have always been identified with Native Americans since the time of the Spanish conquistadores. They were present when the Pilgrims landed at Plymouth Rock and were greeted by some of the friendly Massachusetts Indians. The Crow people have long relied upon these two important food sources for maintaining health and recovering from illness of some sort.

"Remember this," Joy reminded me one day during my "crash course" in Crow diet and medicine, "*never* waste anything! That is what my grandmother taught me and what most Crow grow up believing." She then showed me how to roast pumpkin seeds. The seeds are scooped out after a pumpkin has been cut open and placed on a tray in the sun to dry. The seeds are then placed in a bowl and just enough sunflower seed oil poured over them to lightly coat them. They are mixed well with the hands or with a wooden spoon. Salt is optional but can be stirred in if so desired. The oiled seeds are spread on a metal tray and put in an oven set to 250° F. Stir occasionally and roast until the seeds have begun to turn brown."

They make great energy snacks as I soon discovered. "We use them quite a bit on those children who we think may have intestinal worms," Joy stated. "My grandmother used pumpkin seeds as an effective deworming medicine."

Her method of drying pumpkin was obviously handed down over a number of generations. "For this either pie pumpkin or hubbard squash may be used," she said. "Pick the vegetables off the vine before the skin is tough. Wash the young pumpkins and slice them into strips or circles as you would slice tomatoes. It is not necessary to remove the seeds at this point because they are not fully developed and are yet tender. Spread the strips or circles on a clean tarp or muslin on a table or drying rack to dry in the sun. Turn the strips over and stir them around often to dry quickly. This may take several days to do. In the evening gather the strips, or cover the drying rack with a piece of plastic sheet to protect from moisture. Continue the drying process the next day. When the pumpkin strips are quite dry, put them in a flour sack and hang in a well-ventilated place to continue to dry thoroughly before storing in an air-tight container.

"To cook up some of these pumpkin strips later on, soak what you need of them until swollen. Then cook in cracked marrow bone broth until they are tender. Mix some wheat flour and water to make a smooth paste, and add to the cooked pumpkin, stirring constantly to prevent lumping. Add 1 tablespoonful of bone marrow fat or butter to taste. The thickening should be [of] medium [consistency]. We give this type of food to young children or elderly people who are skinny and in need of something that is filling and nutritious. We say in Crow that 'pumpkin [and squash] are filling-out foods' ; they put pounds on you and give nourishment that sustains. This is always the preferred food among Crow healers for any kind of stomach or bowel problems."

Several other root vegetables occurring in the wild that have been Crow food-medicine favorites for a long time are sego lily, wild potato, wild carrot, wild rhubarb, and bitterroot. Here are the methods for preparing each one of these and the health conditions for which they best apply.

SEGO LILY/MARIPOSA LILY *(Calochortus nuttallii).* "The Crow name is 'Burned on Top of Head,'" Joy mentioned with a smile. "The bulbs of this plant are dug when the flower is in full bloom. The bulbs are sweet and have a very pleasant, creamy taste and flavor. The outer covering or skin is removed when they are to be eaten. The bulbs can be boiled in cracked marrow bone stock or plain stream or well water and thickened as some of the other food plants that I've mentioned to you before. Or they may be eaten fresh. The bulbs are good for those who've suffered starvation or can't eat normal foods."

WILD POTATO *(Claytonia lanceolata).* "We call this one 'mealy root' in the Crow tongue. It is an early spring vegetable ready for use when the white or pink blossoms are in bloom. Mealy root grows where it is moist under brush and along creeks. In the mountains these plants grow in a thick carpet in the clearing where the snow has just melted. The root or bulb grows to the size of a small walnut, [has] dark skin, and creamy-white, mealy meat. The roots are dug, cleaned and cooked in boiling water, mashed and thickened with wheat flour, and sweetened with a little honey to taste. This food is particularly good to overcome an acid stomach and prevent nausea and vomiting."

WILD CARROTS *(Perideridia gairdneri).* I watched as my hostess made some root patties from this vegetable gathered right out of Mother's Nature own hill-and-meadow supermarket "produce section." After sampling one of them, I pronounced it as being better than anything similar I'd ever tasted made with store-bought carrots. "We call this vegetable 'forked grass' or 'squaw root,'" she said. It also goes by the name of yampa.

"This plant grows anywhere there is grass, in open fields, near water, or on tops of the highest hills and mountains. The roots grow either in clusters or form a single root, the size of a young carrot. The skin is rather thick and dark, the meat is cream-color[ed], and crunchy to eat like celery and sweet when fresh. The root is ready when the plant is in bloom. A shovel is the instrument used to dig the roots after a rain, as the ground is soft and yields easily. After washing the roots to remove the sand and dirt, the carrots are boiled until tender. Like the turnip these are mashed by hand, but the food chopper is the quickest way to grind or mash carrots. They may be frozen or dried.

"To prepare, soak the amount desired in warm water, cover the dried vegetable, and let it stand until soft. More cracked marrow bone broth or water may be added to replace the amount the vegetables soaked up. This vegetable needs to be boiled only a short time because it is already cooked. Mix some wheat flour and water to make a paste and add to the carrots to make a medium thick mixture. Add a tablespoonful of bone marrow, or butter and sweeten to taste with some honey.

"This is how you make the wild carrot patties. Wash and cover the carrots with water. Boil until tender, then drain the water and let the vegetable cool. Remove the skin and mash the carrots like potatoes, sweeten just enough to taste and make patties. Fry in butter to brown on both sides. Serve warm. This vegetable tastes more like parsnips than carrots when prepared this way. It can also be baked with mashed sweet potato. This is a wonderful food remedy for pregnant mothers during their 'morning sickness' periods when they can't eat much of anything else. It is also used sometimes with those who are too sick to eat anything else or have no appetite for anything."

WILD RHUBARB (Hercaleum lanatum).   "We call this plant 'Like Skinny Ones,'" she replied. "Botanists call it cow parsnip. Unlike the vegetables that I've already mentioned and you've recorded, the rhubarb is not edible once it is in bloom. It grows along creeks near the mountains. The hollow hairy stalks grow in a cluster, topped by big wide leaves, hairy on the under sides. It has a strong flavor. A taste for this has to be acquired over time.

"The young shoots are best for eating in early spring when they are tender and of less pungent flavor. To dry the wild rhubarb, cut or chop the stalks in lengths of 1 inch and steam them in a small amount of water until quite tender. More water may be added if necessary to prevent scorching. Drain the excess water and spread the cooked vegetable on a clean piece of canvas or muslin on a table in the sun. Cover it with cheese cloth to protect it from flies and stir often to hasten the drying process. When quite dry, store it in a flour sack and hang it up in a well-ventilated place for a few days to be sure all moisture is dried out before storing in airtight containers.

"To prepare, soak one or two of the dried vegetables in warm water or cracked marrow bone stock to cover and let stand until it has taken up the liquid and is plump. Then add more liquid or stock and let it simmer for 10 to 15 minutes. Mix ¼ cup wheat flour with a little water to make a smooth, thin paste. Add this to the simmering vegetables and stir vigorously to prevent lumps. Add 1 tablespoon[ful] of bone marrow fat or suet and let the rhubarb continue to simmer until the thickening is thoroughly cooked, 4 or 5 minutes. This should be a medium thickening. Serve sweetened with some honey.

The fresh vegetable is cut in 1-inch pieces, covered with water or cracked marrow bone stock, cooked in a saucepan until tender, then thickened as above. This has a very delicate, green color and is quite tasty. It is the first, fresh edible vegetable to come up in the spring.

"The Crow have used this as long as I can remember as a tonic for rejuvenating the entire body. It promotes appetite in those not inclined to eat very much. And is a very good astringent for all cases of diarrhea. It is also a useful purgative in its place."

BITTERROOT *(Lewisia rediviva).* "This is our state flower of the Big Sky Country," Joy said with obvious delight. "The Crow name given it means 'bushy root.' It is dug during flower time when the cuticle is easily removed. The white root is dried in the sun until it becomes quite brittle. To prepare, the roots are steeped and soaked in warm water until they are swollen and plump. Then they are drained and boiled in fresh water 2 or 3 times to remove the bitter taste. The roots are swollen to 2 or 3 times the[ir] original size in this process.

The last cooking liquid is either marrow bone stock or plain water. The stock always gives the best flavor. Thicken the stew with a small amount of flour and mix to make a thin paste. Add a small chunk of marrow or suet (about 1 or 2 tablespoonsful) and sweeten to taste with some honey."

The Story of Pemmican—Wonderful Indian Nourishment

Of all the Native American foods ever made, none is so wonderful and sustaining as pemmican. During my two-week visit with Joy Toineeta, I virtually subsisted on this on those days we went into the nearby foothills and mountains to dig for food/medicinal roots and gather other useful herbs.

Pemmican was a common travel food of many Native Americans in Canada, the United States, and Mexico. Slices of lean venison (deer or elk) or buffalo meat were sun dried, pounded to a paste, and packed with melted fat in rawhide bags. Dried currants or wild berries were sometimes included in the paste. Ross Cox spoke of it in his book, mentioning that some of the Pacific Coast Indians in the Northwest used similar fish compounds, usually made from salmon.

Making pemmican is now pretty much a lost art, even among present-day Native Americans. Joy told me one day as I watched and participated with her in its preparation, "Not even my part-Cherokee children or grandchildren are interested in having me teach them how to make this. They say it's easier to go to the Agency store and buy it already made from the white man. It's funny how I'm teaching you, a white man of all people, how we make this, when it should be my own family here watching this."

Fortunately for myself and the readers of this book, I not only witnessed it with my eyes and helped to make some pemmican with my own hands, but I had the good sense to bring along a tape recorder and let it run while my kind hostess gladly shared information and techniques obviously passed on from many previous generations.

"Pemmican is still one of the very special foods in the Crow diet, although there are fewer and fewer of us left who still know how to make it. Grandmothers and mothers carried a supply of pemmican for their lunch on their daily marches in the old days. It was not necessary to stop to prepare a meal while the tribe was on the move. Each warrior took a supply when he joined a war party. This eliminated the necessity of a campfire that would reveal the hiding place of the party to the enemy.

"There is a story that has been handed down from the old days about a couple who left the main camp to get a supply of meat. Their camp was concealed by trees along the creek so they felt quite safe. One day the mother made some pemmican to take on their trip back to the main camp. It took longer than she had planned. Her son who was about three years old pestered his mother for bits of handout while he played around the campfire.

"The husband watched his little son while he played. The boy asked his mother for more pemmican, so she formed a small-size ball and gave it to him and he went outside. Soon he returned without his pemmican and asked for more. The mother gave him another small ball. Again he flew out the door to return later empty-handed. The father watched his son's movements and became curious and alarmed. The next time the boy asked for pemmican, his mother was about to question him when her husband quietly nudged her and said, 'Give him a big ball of pemmican this time. He is not eating any of the handouts you gave him before. And he is not just running out with it.'

"So she made a generous serving and handed it to her son, who was delighted to take it out of the lodge. Soon he returned in the arms of an enemy scout. The father quickly sat up and motioned his visitor to the seat of honor in their lodge and instructed his wife to prepare a quick meal.

"While the wife went about her duty, the men visited by signs. The enemy scout told his host that he and his family were surrounded by a war party. And that he the visitor was posted near the camp to watch and to relay information on their movements and to count the number of men in camp before they attacked. When he came near the lodge to hide in the underbrush to spy, the small boy saw him and came out to share his pemmican.

"The enemy scout said, 'I was very hungry and your son shared his pemmican with me. He has touched my heart so I am going to give you time to escape. First, give every appearance by your activity that you are not aware of the enemy's presence. Build a fire, collect a little kindling, and go after some water. Then as soon as I leave, crawl out of your lodge and go down to the creek and follow the bank downstream until you reach a washout.

"'You will be far enough away and out of sight of the watchful party here. Get out in the open and run for the highest hill to hide and watch until nightfall to continue your journey home. I will lead our war party up the stream and away from you. Before you go, leave your best suit of clothes for me behind the curtain by the entrance. Run as soon as I leave.' And he departed.

"By this time the wife had served her guest and had packed the pemmican, her sewing and tanning tools, and was ready to leave. As soon as the scout finished eating, the host piled more wood on the fire while his wife went for water and collected a little kindling and secured the entrance flap. Then one by one the family crawled out of the shelter to the creek and down the bank. The mother put her child on her back and tied a strip of buckskin around him to her shoulders to free her arms so she could support herself as she felt her way along the bank.

"The three hardly breathed as they quietly picked their way along the bottom of the bank. They finally came to the washout and took a deep breath of air, climbed out, and ran for the hills. They ran as they never ran before. The little family climbed the highest hill to hide along the rocks and kept watch over the surrounding country. They remained hidden there until nightfall then continued their journey home. The scout led the war party in the opposite direction and kept his promise."

Making Pemmican

"My grandmother taught me the art of this," Joy commenced. "Every year that some of our elderly die that means a few less Crow of the older generation who remember how to make pemmican. One day, very soon, there won't be any of us left and the art will be lost for good.

"Take the tenderloin from deer, elk, or beef. The tenderloin is the back strap, a long muscle on each side of the backbone.

"After the carcass has been skinned, use a sharp knife to cut through the tough gristle-like hide over the backbone from the neck to the hipbone and to the ribs. Cut down next to the backbone to the ribs, the full length of the back and remove the long straps from each side of the backbone.

"The tough gristle-like skin on the tenderloin is the sinew used for sewing. To remove the sinew for sewing purposes, remove the outer skin and fat by hand or knife. Next to the tenderloin is a white gristle covering the meat. Use a thin sharp knife to peel this white gristle-like cover carefully, beginning from the wide end of the long tenderloin. Then soak the sinew in water until the meat and fat adhering to the sinew scrapes off easily. Remove all trace of meat and fat, wash the sinew clean, and spread it out smoothly on a flat surface to dry. When dry, it will become loose from the flat surface. Store until needed.

"After removing the sinew, the tenderloin is ready to be sliced and dried. Take the long tenderloin and cut down the center the full length to within one-half inch of cutting through. Then carefully slice the meat away from this center, cut[ting] one side at a time to make a thin sheet of meat, one-inch thick. Handle carefully as this is very tender and will tear apart.

"Spread the sheet of meat on a drying rack or pole, or a window screen that permits the air to dry the meat from the underside. Turn the meat often to hasten drying. It is best to dry the meat on a breezy day. The meat must be quite dry. To make the best pemmican, use [only] tenderloin. However, other dried meat can be used, but remove all visible traces of gristle and connective tissues before roasting in the oven. This makes the pounding and pulverizing process easier.

"Fresh ground lean meat can be used by dry-roasting it. Put the ground meat in a roaster or shallow bread pan and roast in a hot oven. Stir often and pour off the drippings until the meat is brown and quite dry. Remove from the pan and proceed with the pounding with hammer or hatchet on clean canvas until the hard kernels are mashed. Measure the pounded meat and place in a large mixing bowl or large dish pan; add stewed chokecherries, marrow bone fat or suet and sugar, and mix well.

"To roast the dried tenderloin or other dried meat, place it on a flat sheet or in a shallow pan and roast in a hot oven at 425 degrees for 10 to 15 minutes. Watch closely as the dried meat scorches easily. Turn once or twice then take out of the oven and sprinkle a little water on the meat on both sides; this makes a moist powder. Break up the larger pieces to convenient grinding size and put through a food grinder or chopper, using the fine blade.

"Thaw out enough frozen ground chokecherries to equal one-half the amount of pounded meat or soak enough dried cherry patties in warm water to equal one-half the amount of meat. The dried cherry patties should disintegrate and take up most of the water. It is best to pour off excess liquid if the mixture is soupy. Then mix with melted marrow fat collected from cracked marrow bones and melt enough lard to equal the amount of cherries. Mix the cherries and fat with the pounded meat, add sugar to taste. Form into oblong balls to fit the palm of the hand. Place in a shallow pan to store in a cool place to set. Serve warm or cold.

"Pemmican is such a special dish that it is sometimes worth a horse in exchange or gifts of wearing apparel and money today. There is a ceremony called the 'Cooked Meat Sing' that features the pemmican as a means of barter; this is a thanksgiving ceremony. The sponsor is usually the one who is especially thankful for an answered prayer or some event. This is also a means of rewarding or paying for the clan uncles' and aunts' prayers for the sponsor's well-being.

"It is the sponsor's duty to decide whom he wants to invite to the sing. He may invite a few or a great many. This depends on the amount of dried meat and chokecherries he has, because he has to prepare six small balls and a very large one for each of his guests. After the list of guests has been decided, the host prepares sticks from the chokecherry tree branches about the size and length of a pencil for each guest.

"This is the formal invitation and the guest is required to bring the stick to the designated place to be admitted. As he delivers the invitation, the sponsor says only, 'I sing for you at such and such a place and time,' and gives the prepared stick to the person. The name of the ceremony is never mentioned. This is one event that must be carried through to the finish no matter what happens. It cannot be postponed or the set time changed in any way or else, it is believed, very bad luck will befall the host and sponsor. So to protect himself, the sponsor does not mention the name of the ceremony as he may not be able to carry out his obligations due to very serious circumstances beyond his control.

"The host selects a man who is known to have strong 'Bear Medicine' or owns a fossil as his medicine and as his protector to conduct the sing.

"As each guest arrives, he returns the stick to the host and is admitted. He takes his place in a circle in the room with his wife. No children are allowed in the ceremony unless parents or grandparents bring a child purposely to seek a clan uncle's blessing or prayers. The clan uncle is given a horse for payment. The clan uncle is then obliged to give the large ball of pemmican in return. No one is allowed to go in or out after the ceremony begins until a certain procedure in the sing is reached and the medicine man grants a recess.

"The host hires the medicine man to conduct the sing and pays him with four articles of some value. The pemmican is placed before this man after the opening prayer and burning of the incense and he distributes the seven pemmican balls to each man, six small ones and one large one. This is the large one that is worth a horse.

"Following the opening prayer, the child [if any] for whom prayers and blessings are sought is admitted and he calls each guest by name and says, 'I sing for you.' The guest is obliged to offer a special prayer for the child or recounts a particularly pleasant dream of a prophetic nature for the child as a way of blessing. He says to the child, 'I will arrive with you safely at this time of the year (a time which is usually in the future).' When a clan uncle or aunt receives a gift at any time, he or she is obliged to recount a dream for the giver and this is considered a blessing or a very special prayer.

"The medicine man begins the sing. After the opening prayer, burning the incense and smudging the medicine bundle, the bundle is passed to the guests. Each guest takes the bundle and holds it to his breast and offers a prayer for the sponsor or for the person for whom the ceremony is conducted until everyone has prayed. The bundle is then placed in the center of the circle. With a rattle to keep time, the sing begins.

"The medicine man sings first and he gives each clan uncle and aunt a ball of pemmican for the privilege of singing. He sings at least four of his medicine and power songs then any number of social or other songs that he particularly likes. The rattle is passed to the next guest and he does the same.

"If he wishes to buy very special prayers or blessings from an uncle, he speaks for his large portion of pemmican and gives him a horse for it. If he does not have a horse, he may give him a sum of money instead. The guests are required to give a gift to the sponsor and this is placed near the medicine bundle. The length of the sing depends on the number of songs each one sings; sometimes it lasts all night."

Plenty-Coups (*Aleek-chea-ahoosh* in Crow, which means Many Achievements), a famous warrior-chieftain, received his name from his grandfather. At the time of his birth in the summer of 1848 near the present site of Billings, Montana, the old man told his parents, "I have dreamed that [your son] shall live to count many coups and be old; my dream also told me that he shall be a chief—the greatest chief our people will ever have." This prophecy was later realized. Plenty-Coups died in 1932.

But during his lengthy reign over the Crow Nation, he stressed the importance of "three necessities" (as he called them) to the life of every Native American: singing, prayer, and pemmican. "To the Crow, song is the breath of the spirit that consecrates the act of life; [for] prayer calls up the helping spirits that our people depend on every day," he once said. As for prayer and the practice of religion, he made this singular observation another time: "The inevitable duty of the Crow is the duty of prayer. [This is] the daily recognition of the Unseen and Supernatural. Whenever a Crow comes upon a scene that is strikingly beautiful or sublime [to him] . . . he pauses for an instant in the attitude of worship. He sees no need for setting apart one day in seven as a holy day, since to him *all* days belong to the Great Spirit." And of pemmican, he stated this in his autobiography: "Pemmican is the great food of all [Indian] nations including the Crow. It is not only the food of life but also of friendship—it sustains and supports whatever it comes in contact with."

Chapter Six

Earth Medicines of the Native Americans

PART II: MATERIA MEDICA OF THE CROW NATION

The Medicine of Her Ancestors

This chapter contains an inventory of medicinal plants and other natural substances which have been used by the Crow Nation in the past for treating a wide variety of ailments. Many of them are readily available on Crow Agency land and commonly grow elsewhere, too. Only a few items are imported and not indigenous to the reservation as such.

I felt highly honored and especially privileged that Joy Yellowtail Toineeta, an expert tribal herbalist in the healing ways of plants, had condescended to share her vast botanical knowledge with me, a white man and an outsider, of all people! "It's probably as it should be," she philosophized one day early on in my two-week stay with her.

Though she was somewhat happy to share her large inventory of herbal information with someone, yet for her it was still done with mixed feelings. A kind of bittersweet joy attended her person as she tried to make the best of a less-than-ideal situation. She didn't blame me for the way she felt, but rather placed it where it properly belonged, namely, to her own family relations "as it should be," she remarked several times. And if that wasn't possible, then certainly to other tribal members. "Indian should be teaching Indian," she insisted, "not Indian teaching white man, as I'm doing with you."

But through it all, we somehow survived our cultural differences, and our mutual respect for each other helped to bridge whatever small gap may have existed between us. Much of this medical lore that was tape-recorded with her permission appears here for the very first time in print. I have sought to present it in pretty much the same way as it was related to me during our many walks in the nearby hills, mountains, and meadows on numerous herb-hunting forays. I believe that by leaving most of it unedited, her unique character and strong personality come through. This is essential for a book such as this, in which the basic "soul" of different folk healers can emerge undisturbed by this author, for the most part. The only thing I undertook to do was to organize this information into a more coherent format for the benefit of readers; otherwise, it's the late Joy Yellowtail Toineeta coming through loud and clear.

"The uses of the plants and natural substances that I will be discussing with you," she began one morning, "were known only to a very selected few at one time. The 'doctors' of the old days guarded their knowledge of plant uses and kept them absolutely secret. It was the custom then as it is today to buy the secret formulas and the techniques. The purchaser was taught and was also sworn to guard the secret techniques and knowledge until he or she was ready to pass it on to a younger person.

"In time many of these became household remedies and practices. The present childhood diseases against which our babies were inoculated were unknown. There were many other diseases that were unheard of such as polio, muscular dystrophy, tuberculosis, smallpox, measles, mumps, and chickenpox. These were regarded as white man's diseases and the Crow children never got them because of the way we ate and lived, staying close to nature at all times as much as we could.

"You will notice, Dr. John, from the plants and substances that I will be showing you, that an inkling of our tribe's health profile will begin to emerge. Crow people were healthier and more robust than they are now. The men grew to immense size as has been observed and recorded by the early explorers, historians, the artists such as George Catlin and others who came in contact with our people. This was a society of 'the survival of the fittest' and they were fit to live a life in the wide open spaces.

"The human body requires proper and balanced nourishment to develop and to grow to the size the Crow men grew to and to remain healthy. Nutrition as we know it today is concerned with balancing the 'Basic Four' [food groups], and how the body utilizes these to function properly. The Crow diet was basically protein balanced by the minerals, vitamins, and carbohydrates of the native fruits (mostly berries) and root vegetables. The natural sugars in the wild fruits were the only known sweeteners. Salt as such was not known to us.

"There was so much physical activity to provide food, clothing, shelter, and living by the chase that no one had time to sit down to become obese or to develop hardening of the arteries. Environmental sanitation was hardly a problem as the tribe was on the move almost daily. Water life was respected to the point of giving a share of one's food with a prayer that the tribe might continue to enjoy an abundance of food and that the 'water people' might help in safe crossing of the larger rivers such as the Yellowstone, Missouri, and Big Horn. Pollution of our streams was impossible with this kind of reverence and respect.

"Personal grooming and cleanliness, as modern man practices it, starts with a bath or a shower, with running hot and cold water. For the Crow Indian a daily bath, winter and summer, was also an absolute must beginning with the camp crier's reveille at the break of dawn. In my early childhood, my grandparents assumed part of the childrearing responsibility. One of my vivid memories is a hole chopped in the ice so each member of the family could take his daily bath no matter what the temperature registered. None of us could read it anyway. I returned to the house many times with frozen braids, but this must have toughened me to ride horseback five miles to school during the winter when I reached school age."

Crow Indian Materia Medica

AMERICAN ELM (*Ulmus americana*). "The Crows say 'balitice' or good wood.' Basic uses were: (1) to check severe nose bleeds and hemorrhages; and (2) to relieve constipation. The inner bark is scraped and boiled. The solution is sniffed into the nostril until bleeding ceases. A strong infusion is prepared as for hemorrhage and taken warm to relieve constipation."

BALSAM FIR (*Abies balsamea*). "Our people used to smear resin from this tree over burns, sores, and cuts, but not so much anymore. My grandmother and I have sometimes applied chunks of this tree gum over the chest or back of some of the men whenever they suffered from pain in the heart or chest. It seems to have given them much relief, which I ascribe to the turpentine in the resin. I have frequently steeped some of the inner bark or liquid resin in hot water as a tea for chest pains and pulmonary troubles. The gum has been taken internally by some of our promiscuous young people to treat venereal diseases, and applied externally for sores resulting from them. The strong turpentine content in a small piece of chewed resin, when mixed with saliva and swallowed, helps to bring up accumulated mucus and effectively clears up lung congestion."

BALSAM NEEDLES (*Tsuga heterophylla*). "This is *bailic-itce* in Crow or 'that which is fragrant' and [it is often combined with] deer's perfume [sex glands] *u:xizba:ilicitce,* for the following uses: (1) for cough and respiratory congestion for babies, also for pneumonia; (2) as a mild laxative for children; (3) for incense. The balsam needles and pieces of the dried sex glands of bucks are best used in the late summer and early fall. Both are dried in the sun. Pieces of the deer glands are then crushed and mixed in equal proportion with the balsam needles and stored in a container. For a cold and cough, it is best to brew enough tea for the day, usually two or three cups. About two pinches of dried sex glands and needle mixture for each cup are sufficient. Heat the water and the needles and gland pieces to a boil, then let steep, strain, and store. It is best to take the tea hot. For a mild laxative, a stronger infusion is prepared as above. Dried balsam needles and pieces of shriveled sex glands from deer are sometimes sprinkled over live coals for incense."

BEAR ROOT (*Lomatium macrocarpum*). "The Crow word *ee:zay* could be translated to mean 'big root.' Bear root was used: (1) to treat coughs and sore throats; (2) to reduce swelling; (3) to purify air as with incense; (4) to relieve colic; (5) as an additive to fertilizer for tobacco planting ceremony; and (6) in healing salve to treat sores. The root is harvested when the plant is in bloom. These are as large as beets and larger. The roots are roasted in a bed of live coals until cooked through then cooled and the burned outer crust is scraped and stored.

"For a cold, shavings from the root are steeped in boiled water with a piece of fat. The infusion is taken hot as needed. For sore throat, a piece of the root is chewed and the juice is swallowed as needed. To treat swelling, a poultice is prepared by boiling shavings of the root in a small amount of water to obtain a strong infusion. Shavings are removed and applied to the swelling and kept saturated with the tea. Ceremonial incense is prepared by scraping or shaving the root and sprinkling it on live coals. This is also used to purify and deodorize air. Shavings of the root are mixed with buffalo chips and sacred tobacco seed for planting. To prepare a salve, pulverized shavings are added and boiled with melted tallow with a small amount of water until the water is boiled off. The congealed fat is stored in a container and used as needed."

BLUE JOINT GRASS (*Agropyron smithii*). "*Bikka:ka:ze* or 'real grass' is known to others as western wheat grass. The tough young blades are used to scrape eyelids to treat trachoma. A strong infusion of the grass tea is a useful eyewash for cataracts."

BOX ELDER (*Acer negundo*). "The Crows call it *bizbe*. Its sap was collected for sweetening, and its branches were used for shinney ball sticks. This tree belongs to the maple family, so like the cottonwood, the sap furnishes a sweet treat when it runs in early spring. A chunk of the wood is chopped out of the horizontal trunk to fill up like a cup. The sap is collected when the cup is full. Box elder does not break easily, so it makes a good ball stick. The natural L-shaped branches make the best shinney sticks. Boil the tree wood down to half its water content and rub the cooled tea over arthritic or rheumatic joints. Tapping box elder trees for sap in the spring was quite a social event for the young people in the olden days. The young people were permitted to tap and to gather the sap. It was a sweet, nourishing drink that everyone enjoyed."

CACTUS (*Opuntia polycantha*). "The Crows say *bickalia,* [while] others call it prickly pear. The juice from the pulpy leaf is applied to painted rawhide surfaces. The clear, sticky juice dried to form an insoluble protective coating. The stickers of the cactus are removed with pliers and the leaf is split to rub on the rawhide surfaces. The sticky juice has also been rubbed on severely chafed skin or over wounds and burns to form a clear, protective coating so dirt and other debris don't get in to cause infection. Red berries from another type of cactus are eaten fresh."

CHEWING GUM. Joy Toineeta philosophized somewhat in connection with this habit as it applied to other traits of her people and the white man. She waxed eloquent in her wise observations and I saw no need to interfere with this pleasant and remarkable distraction. "Emerging from the nomadic stone age to the first encounter with the white man, the Crow Indian found a people from an entirely different world. The Indian stepped back to watch for an explanation and an understanding of these strangely behaved people. The sound of that clash of the first head-on collision of these two cultures has grown in volume to the present time in more than the gum-chewing area.

"We speak glibly today of the transition and finally assimilation into the white man's world. We even applaud the individual who seems to have made the grade. If the truth were known, there is not a Crow Indian who is comfortable in his own society who wishes to lose his identity. Those who have lost their tribal customs are the successful ones to become integrated and assimilated. These are the 'white' Indians. Even they, in many cases, have to keep their Indian blood a secret to remain integrated or assimilated unless they are successful and influential enough in whatever field they are established to boast of their great-grandfather's Indian great-grandmother.

"Those who are in a position to see some of the detrimental changes are saddened by the loss of some of the finer aspects of their tribal life and organization. For instance, the changes that have affected the very strict personal discipline that was quite adequate for the individual may be detrimental. Without discipline in his personal, religious, and family life, the Crow Indian was not considered a man.

"There were established tribal protocols, social graces, personal etiquette, and conduct based on a way of life and need. Many of these are in direct conflict with Emily Post and Amy Vanderbilt, so that even today we find a constant hammering and erosion of what is left to conform to the mold that our own Indian benefactors believe to be the only way we will succeed as a people.

"There is a need to mention these conflicts only in passing here. Now to go to a lesser one in the habit of gum chewing. This personal habit has become naturally acceptable. In early Emily Post time it was not.

"Gum chewing had a function in the Crow culture. The native gum was not a product of the tropical tree from which Wrigley's spearmint and others on the market are made. The sources of our gum were the white pine *(Pinus monticola)* from the hardened resin collected from the trunk of the trees and from a species of milkweed *(Lygodesmia juncea)*. [The latter] was pulled up by the roots and exposed to the sun until the milk that oozed out dried and congealed to a rubbery substance. Hundreds of plants had to be uprooted to collect the congealed milk but it was done. One had to be careful not to expose the resin gum to fresh air while chewing or it became granulated and it had to be chewed all over again. If these two substances were chewed long enough, they softened somewhat and could be popped noisily.

"I never knew of a young person—mostly the young women—

who ever got gum disease or cavities if they faithfully chewed on the tree gum and milkweed latex long enough. Sometimes these well-masticated substances would be removed from someone's mouth and affixed to an open wound or bad sore or nasty burn of some kind. These afflictions would heal more quickly when this 'Indian gum' was put on them.

"The elders used to tell us that this gum popping was an accepted practice for a young woman in the old days. She chewed daintily and popped her gum demurely, if one could accomplish such a feat. To attract the attention of the opposite sex was one practice in particular. She was not allowed to attract or draw attention to herself otherwise in any boisterous manner or dress. She was taught to move and speak softly and to always conduct herself with dignity and in a manner that would not cause any embarrassment to the men of her family.

"A man, on the other hand, was allowed to dress in his finest clothes and trappings, to ride his fanciest mount, and to openly sing and flirt with the ladies. Chewing and popping the tough pine resin and the rubbery milkweed substances was certainly a small leeway to the young woman to let the world know that she was around! So we continue to chew and pop gum at social functions, on the streets, in school, on campus, in church, and everywhere on the reservation. But now most of us prefer the white man's manufactured gum compared to the healthier alternatives our parents and grandparents chewed."

CLAYS. "Red and white clay are mineral deposits in the earth and have been very useful to the Crow. The finely sifted red powder mixed with fat is the best and quickest healing salve for diaper burns and heat rash in the summer. Usually one or two applications are sufficient. The red salve is also very good for athlete's foot. Severe wind burns and chap and sunburns also heal quickly when the red salve is applied.

"White clay, a fine white powder, mixed with water checks diarrhea. This is also used to clean and whiten buckskin. A wet paste is first rubbed in the soiled spot and left to dry. It is then scraped off with the rough edge of an instrument or sandpaper till clean."

COFFEE (*Coffea arabica*). The coffee tree, actually a small evergreen with smooth, ovate leaves and clusters of fragrant white flowers that mature into deep red fruits about a half-inch long, is native to Ethiopia, where it was known before 1000 A.D. Varieties of this species are important cash crops in many countries, especially in South America and East Africa. Brazil is the leading producer. The United States imports 80 percent of this coffee species.

The variety of recipes and prescriptions for roasting, brewing, and serving coffee reflect the diversity of consumer tastes and cultural preferences. Coffee owes its popularity in part to the stimulative effect of its caffeine content. The deeply crimson coffee berries, commonly called "cherries," contain between 1.5 to 3.2 percent caffeine; other xanthine alkaloids include theobromine and theophylline, but in trace amounts only.

"In the beginning our people knew nothing of this substance," Joy Toineeta said. "But once the early fur trappers introduced this brew to the Abasorkee war parties or scouts who had occasion to meet and share their fare, it won their immediate approval. And while the Crow have consistently consumed coffee for mostly its beverage status, it has also been used by some of our healers as a medicinal drink for pulmonary disorders. Consumption of the lungs, pneumonia, colds which settle in the chest, and accumulated mucus in the breathing passages have all been treated with hot, boiled, black coffee, sipped slowly. Some white people who have suffered from asthma or bronchitis have even been helped by this Crow remedy; they told us afterwards how much better they were able to breathe following a hot cup of coffee. So while it is definitely a white man's beverage, the Crow Indians have used it to their own good advantage.

"My grandmother was fond of telling this true story, which she witnessed as a child with her own mother. During their wandering and following the game along the foothills of the Big Horn Mountains, one day some of the Crow warriors who smoked and visited with white trappers remarked among themselves about how delicious and revivifying the wonderful hot brew was which they had been given to drink when they shared a meal with the others. They all

expressed their desire for another taste. Now this aroused the curiosity of some of the other braves who remained in camp and overheard
this discussion and hadn't as yet tasted it for themselves. They, too,
became desirous of trying some of the trappers' much-talked-about
brew. So it was decided that the camp would move to the Elk River
trading post to trade pelts for the articles that had become necessary.
The men mentioned rifles and ammunition. The blacksmith who ham-
mered sheets of copper and bronze into pots, pans, water buckets, and
axes was mentioned, as also were the beads and calico that the
women needed. So early the next morning the camp was on the move
for these purported reasons, when in fact it was really for another cup
of coffee.

"In a few days the tribe arrived at the trading post. Teepees were
set up, kindling was gathered, and the lodges were made comfortable.
There was an air of excitement as each family prepared the bundles of
fur pelts for barter. At last when everyone was ready, the women
packed their bundles on their backs and left for the post. The trading
began in earnest. Some traded for brass buckets and kettles; others
traded for calico, beads, and trinkets. The men spent their time at the
rifle and ammunition department. The smithy was busy forging
knives, awls, and other equipment that was needed. The man who
started this long trek for his cup of coffee bought his bag of green coffee beans and rushed home with his wife. He passed on to his wife the
instructions he was given on their preparation. He said, 'Roast these
seeds slowly in the fire until they are good and brown. Then grind
them and have it ready for my evening meal when I return from my
hunt.'

"The anxious wife listened carefully to avoid any mistakes in the
preparation of these strange seeds that she traveled so far to taste. As
soon as her husband left, she built a big roaring fire, then let it die
down on a bed of coals. She opened the bag of coffee beans and scattered them on the coals and stirred them around until they were
roasted quite brown. Then she separated the coals from the coffee
beans. She did not forget that her husband told her to grind them. She
took out her grinding stones from one of her parfleche bags and did a
wonderful job of grinding.

"That evening when the husband returned to his camp he announced that he was ready for the coffee first, for he had thought of little else all day save that as he hunted with the rest of the men. The wife happily announced that it was quite ready for him to try. She pulled out the rawhide bag that she used to store her food and took out handfuls of something and placed it in the wooden serving plate and handed it to her husband. It was the ground coffee all right, but with chunks of animal fat mixed in! The husband asked, 'What is this?'

"She replied that it was the coffee prepared exactly as he instructed her that morning before he left. She added, 'It did not taste very good alone so I added the chunks of fat and we all thought it was quite delicious after that.'

"The husband was so disgusted he could not say a word but he gave her such a look that only a wife could know the meaning of it. When he regained his composure he told her that it was not to be eaten that way, it was to be boiled in water like meat! The poor, confused wife jumped up and said cheerfully, 'Why did you not say so in the first place? Here, let me fix it right for you.' And this she did, much to his regret!

"She took the coffee and fat mixture and poured it into the kettle of meat that she had prepared for their evening meal and set the kettle back on the fire. When it boiled and turned a dirty, greasy, brown color, she happily brought it to her husband and poured him a full bowl. By this time the husband had lost his appetite for the meat and the coffee that had obsessed him all day long. Who could drink this dirty, greasy brew anyway, he muttered to himself. He stood up, kicked over the whole kettle, and stomped out of their lodge in a great huff.

"This turned out to be a terribly expensive and very painful experience for the poor wife, my grandmother said, but she eventually learned to brew a good cup of coffee after all!"

COTTONWOOD (*Populis sargentii*). "This is *bahkuzua* in the Crow tongue and is translated to 'green seed pods.' It is used for sweetening and firewood. In the spring of the year when the cotton flies, the bark of the cottonwood is ready to yield the sweet inner bark. This becomes a great social occasion for the young people, one of the few times a young man could openly court his lady of choice. With other couples, the young people were allowed to enter the woods to search and select the trees, to debark them and scrape the inner bark to collect the sweet sap to bring home to share with other members of the family. The other use was for firewood. The dry wood gives a clean, hot fire and it is plentiful. It is a soft wood so it was not difficult for the women who gathered wood to break it up into convenient loads and to pack it home on their backs.

The other source of natural sweeteners for the Crow was the tender, juicy inner bark of the cottonwood tree. In the spring when the cotton on the trees burst and was flying, it was a sign to us that the natural sugar in the sap was at its peak. Our medicine men and women would gather some in a pail to take back to their lodges and store away until it was needed as a remedy. They treated sour stomachs in infants and young children and older adults by mixing a little of the cottonwood sap in a small amount of hot water and then giving it to their patients to drink. This is also good for relieving heartburn and stomach gas, as I have used it many times myself on others for these problems. The mouth could also be rinsed with a little sap in some warm water to get rid of halitosis.

FRAGRANT YELLOW BLOSSOMS (*Matricaria matricarioides*). "The Crow word for this is *ba:uhpazi:lilicitce,* meaning 'fragrant yellow blossoms.' The buds and leaves were collected, dried and crushed to line baby cradles with. It had a wonderful calming effect on restless infants, who would cease their wiggling around and fall to sleep almost immediately."

HONEYSUCKLE PLANT. "Grandmothers instructed the children in their charge on the sources of edible plants, and how to utilize them. Sugar as such was not known then. Only the natural sources were then available to us. In the spring when the flowers are in bloom, there is a species of wild honeysuckle (*Lonicera* species) with lots of flowers. Groups of children would go out to gather flowers from it, while the parents were engaged in shinny games or others sports like horse races, or enjoying an outing for a picnic. When there was a supply large enough to permit the children to sit down to enjoy it, they did just that. Each would get and then pull out the individual white blossoms in the stem that resembled blue bells and suck the nectar from it. This was quite sweet and had a very pleasant flavor."

HORSE MINT (*Monarda fistulosa*).   "The Crow name is *bah-puize*. It is used for respiratory congestion, for colds and cough, and for the flu. A strong infusion is prepared from stems, leaves, and blossoms, strained, and taken hot for colds and coughs, as often as necessary. The plant is harvested in bloom, dried in the sun, and stored in airtight containers."

HORSE SCENT.   "This is the warty growth on the foreleg of a horse [which] is boiled in a small amount of water. The tea or broth is then given to quicken labor in childbirth. It causes the cervix to dilate for a quick and easy birth."

HUCKLEBERRY (*Gaylussacia*).   "The wild huckleberry plant is used to brew a beverage like peppermint. The leaves and stems are dropped into boiling water until the desired color of tea is obtained. This is like the modern black tea and is very good. Serve it hot or cold."

JOINT WEED/VARIEGATED HORSETAIL (*Equisetum variegatum*).   "It is called 'ghost's pipe' or *ahpala:sizipcikizze* by the Crows. This plant is harvested in the blossom stage. The tip of the plant is velvety brown when it is ready. These are dried in the sun and stored for use. It is used: (1) as a diuretic, and (2) to relieve pain in the bladder and prostate area. For man or beast for failure to void, a strong infusion is prepared by boiling the jointed weed in water, straining, and taking the infusion hot as often as needed until relieved. To relieve pain, a hot poultice is prepared from the strained plant and applied to the lower abdomen. The hot solution is used to keep the poultice saturated."

JUNIPER (*Juniperus scopulorum*).   "This tree is often called cedar by others, while we Crow know it as *bukuxbe* or 'holy' or 'medicine wood.' Its uses are intended: (1) to stop hemorrhages; (2) to induce appetite and settle upset stomach; (3) for incense; (4) to check diarrhea; and (5) to cleanse and heal a woman after childbirth. To stop lung or nose hemorrhage, shavings from cedar wood are boiled in water, strained, and given to drink as needed. The infusion is also sniffed into the nostrils until bleeding ceases. To settle an upset stomach, two or three berries are chewed and swallowed at intervals until the desired effect is obtained. To induce appetite, one or two berries are chewed and swallowed a short time before a meal. For ceremonial incense, dried leaves are sprinkled over live coals. To check diarrhea, an infusion is prepared from boiling the needles in water, straining, and giving after each bowel movement. This same infusion is given after a birth for cleansing and healing."

KINNIKINNICK (*Arctostaphylos uva-ursi*). "The Crow name is *o:pi:zia,* which means 'mixed with tobacco.' Its uses include the following: (1) as a smoking mixture; (2) as a treatment for canker sores in the mouth; (3) as a treatment for open sores; and (4) for nourishment. This plant does not grow high. It clings to the ground and forms a thick carpet. The branches are broken to harvest the leaves. The leaves are dried in the sun and used for pipe smoking. Dried leaves are pulverized and the powder is applied to canker sores in the mouth. An open sore is cleansed and the leaf powder is sprinkled over it. In midsummer when the berries are bright red, they are edible."

I enjoyed some of this kinnikinnick in an old calumet (a highly ornamented ceremonial pipe) one evening which had been in Joy's family for a long time. I found it a most pleasant smoking experience. This event followed a very rich dinner of beaver tail stew, which had to be boiled for a long time on account of its toughness. The onions, potatoes, and wild carrots (akin to parsnips) added to the flavor. She served it with some buckskin bread and chokecherry tea—"a *real* Crow Indian dinner," she insisted.

LICHEN AND WILLOW FORMULA (*Evernia vulkina*)/ (*Salix amygdaloides*). "Lichen in Crow is *awizce* or 'ground rust,' and willow is *bili:ce.* The willow bark and lichen are boiled together for an eyewash solution for removal of cataracts. This is used as needed. The lichen [itself] is parched, pulverized, and sprinkled on canker sores. A tea made from the lichen is used to gargle for laryngitis and also as a mouthwash for canker sores. Lichen is chewed to prevent cavities. The green lichen on pine trees *(ba:i:zi:le)* in translation describes the yellow dyeing qualities of this fungi. It is used as incense to quicken labor in childbirth and as ceremonial incense."

"LIKE COMB"/ECHINACEA (*Echinacea angustifolia*). "Harvesting of this plant's roots takes place when it is in bloom; they are washed and dried in the sun. For a cold, a piece of root is kept in the mouth and the juice slowly swallowed. For a toothache, a piece of the root is softened in the mouth and held to the offending tooth. An infusion is made by crushing or breaking the dried root into small pieces and boiling it in water. This is strained and given in small amounts until colic pains are relieved."

As a historical side note apart from what Joy said about this herb, the following data from Melvin R. Gilmore's *Uses of Plants by the Indians of the Missouri River Region* (Washington, D.C.: Government Printing Office, 1919; 33rd Annual Report of the Bureau of American Ethnology) may prove interesting to all those who are acquainted with echinacea in some way: "It was said that [Indian] jugglers [medicine men involved solely in disease diagnoses] bathed their hands and arms in the juice of this plant so that they could take out a piece of meat from a boiling kettle with the bare hand without suffering pain, to the wonderment of onlookers. A Winnebago said he had often used the plant to make his mouth insensible to heat, so that for show he could take a live coal into his mouth. Burns were bathed with the juice to give relief from the pain, and the plant was used in the steam bath to render the great heat endurable." I personally have used *fresh* echinacea in poultice form to treat severe burns with good success on two different occasions!

MULLEIN (*Verbascum thapsus*). This common meadow weed, easily identified by its furry leaves, grows in many places on Crow Agency land. Joy Toineeta explained that the leaves were sometimes smoked like tobacco for the relief of asthma, bronchitis, and sore throat. And when the boiled root was sweetened, it could be given to children suffering from croup. Sometimes mullein roots were dug up, cleaned of their dirt, and boiled with the roots of button willow for an internal drink for severe coughs. A smoke smudge has sometimes been made in the past of the leaves and the fumes then inhaled for autumnal catarrh (hay fever) or sinusitis, as well as to revive an unconscious patient.

NEW GROWTH OF YOUNG WILLOW (*Salix* species).   "The Crow word is *bili:ce,* for which there is no translation," Joy said. "An infusion from the crushed root of the new or young willow is used for scalp treatment for falling hair. Willow bark is chewed to clean teeth, to prevent cavities, and to relieve headaches."

NEZ PERCÉ ROOT (*Angelica* species).   "Often this plant is called wild celery root. It is used (1) as an additive to smoking tobacco; (2) as incense; (3) for sinus infections; (4) for sore throats; colds and coughs; and (5) for earaches and abscessed ears. This is not a native plant but it has become so useful that the Crow Indians traded for it from their Nez Perce friends in Idaho and Washington states. Shavings of this root added to kinnikinnick and tobacco make wonderful smoking. Shavings sprinkled on live coals produce a fine incense. Shavings are added to boiling water for a steam inhalant for sinus infection and congestion. A strained strong infusion made from mashed roots and boiling water is sniffed into the nostrils. A piece of root is kept in the mouth and the juice is swallowed for a sore throat. For a cold and cough, a strong infusion is taken as needed. One or two drops of the warm, strong infusion is dropped in the ear for an earache. For an abscessed ear, a poultice from the shavings is applied to the affected area."

PEPPERMINT (*Mentha arvensis*).   "The Crow name is *shu-shu-ah*. A literal translation in Crow is 'spit, spit.' Perhaps this has reference to the strong, biting taste of the mint. It has many uses, for example, as a (1) calming beverage; (2) nerve tonic and diuretic; (3)

treatment for swelling; (4) favorite snakebite remedy; and (5) wonderful flavoring for pounded meat.

"For a nice beverage, pick a handful of stems and leaves from some fresh plants and wash them before dropping them into boiling water. Let them steep until the tea is the desired color. The tea can be used hot or iced. For winter uses, pick, wash, and dry the stems and leaves in the sun. Pack in airtight containers and use as needed like you would any other herbal tea.

"An infusion stronger than for beverage is brewed for the tonic and diuretic effects of this plant. Several cups of the hot tea are taken during the day. A strong infusion is made from leaves and stems. They are then removed to be applied to a swelling and the tea is used to keep the poultice saturated until the swelling is reduced.

"There are two mint combinations for treatment of snakebites. One method is to take equal parts of peppermint leaves and stems, sagebrush (*Artemisia* species), and buffalo perfume (*Madia glomerata*) and boil them to make a strong solution. The plants are removed afterwards to apply to the wound after it has been bled and cleansed with some of the tea. The poultice is kept saturated with the heated solution. This is repeated with fresh poultices and solution until the swelling is reduced. The second method involves making a solution from a combination of mint and chewing tobacco. The mint and tobacco are used for the poultice to reduce the swelling and to draw the poison and infection out. The solution is kept as hot as the patient can stand and applied until the swelling is reduced.

"Mint leaves are added for flavoring meat. After dried, roasted, or jerked meat has been crushed or pulverized, a few crushed leaves of mint are added and mixed thoroughly and stored in a container for a day or so to improve the flavor of the meat."

PEYOTE (*Lophophora williamsii*). "The Crow word is *bickalia,* which is the same word for cactus, for this plant belongs to the cactus family. Peyote is not native to the Crow Agency lands. It grows in southern Texas and Mexico and is used to treat many ailments. But Crow medicine men and women have used it specifically in easing the labor pains of women in childbirth. One or two buttons are chewed and swallowed when a pregnant woman is about to deliver."

PUFF BALLS (*Lycoperdon* species).   "The Crow word for this is *I:wa:izdalete,* a translation of which is 'used to make one blind.' The black powder in the puff ball is used to treat impetigo or open sores. The sores are cleansed and the powder is sprinkled over them. The powder has also been sprinkled on infant skin in cases of diaper rash. And as a prophylactic and therapeutic measure, Crow medicine men and women used to place puffballs on the navels of newborns and leave them there until the withered remains of the cords fell off. The spores or pulverized heads of puff balls were once used as hemostatics to stop hemorrhages. Puff ball powder was packed into the wounds of body cavities."

RED DOGWOOD (*Cornus stolonifera*).   "Translation of the Crow name *bili:zi:zze* for this is 'red willow.' Its bark is used for smoking, and the white berries (1) serve as an additive to the fertilizer for tobacco seed planting, or (2) are chewed to dissolve tartar deposits on teeth. For smoking, the outer red bark is carefully peeled off and the second layer is scraped down to the wood and dried thoroughly in the sun. It is then mashed or broken into a coarse powder or particles and mixed with dried kinnikinnick, or broken coarsely fine and added in equal parts to twisted tobacco leaves. A little wild celery root shaving is added to this mixture to give off a wonderful aroma. For fertilizer, the white berries are added to the prepared buffalo chips mixed with the sacred seeds, moistened, and dropped into the prepared ground. To remove the tartar deposit on teeth, handfuls of the bitter berries are chewed, some of the juice being swallowed."

ROOT THAT TURNS BACK (*Polygonum bistortoides*).   "The tiny, white, turned-back tips of the root of this plant are chewed raw for correcting diarrhea."

ROSE BUSH ROOT (*Rosa* species).   "The Crow name for this is *bickapapa:li:cihcizia* and is used in the following ways: (1) to check diarrhea; (2) to reduce swelling; (3) to check nose and mouth hemorrhage; and (4) to relieve sore throat and tonsillitis. To check diarrhea, the root is washed, crushed, and boiled in water and the infusion is given after each bowel movement. To reduce swelling, the same infusion is used for hot compresses until the swelling goes down. For hemorrhage of the nose and mouth, tonsillitis, and sore throat, a strong infusion is prepared. It is sniffed up into the nostril until the bleeding stops. For hemorrhage from the mouth, the infusion is taken by mouth until relief is obtained. For tonsillitis and sore throat, the infusion is used to gargle with and some is swallowed."

ROSIN WEED (*Grindelia squarrosa*). "The Crow name for this plant is 'stink yellow blossom,'" Joy Toineeta mentioned. "It is called rosin or gypsum weed or curlcup gumweed and is harvested when blossoms have formed the curlcup. They are dried and stored. Uses include the treatment of (1) cough and catarrh, (2) after-birth pains, and (3) swelling. They are also used as an incense to dispel evil spirits. An infusion is prepared from the blossom ends of the plant. The hot tea is taken as needed for cough. The same tea is sniffed into the nostrils for catarrh. Hot tea is taken after a baby is born to prevent or lessen the after pain. Hot compresses from the strong infusion are applied to reduce swelling. To dispel evil spirits, crushed blossom ends are sprinkled over live coals, and the whole house or lodge is smudged."

SACHETS. "The fragrance of leaves and blossoms appealed to the Crow men and women as it does to people everywhere. It was possible to dry some so they retained their fragrance. To use, a little of the dried plants was moistened to apply to the hair, body, or clothing. A drop or so of oil from beaver castor [obtained from scent glands in an anal pouch] was sometimes added in some mixtures.

"The ingredients in the best sachets and perfumes were kept secret. One that is commonly known is a blend of three or four plants. These are horse mint blossoms (*Monarda fistulosa*), the plant that is called 'smells like willows' *(Ivesia gordonii),* and seeds from a plant that grows in the lower altitudes along the rivers called 'rough-end seed' *(Thalictrum dasycarpum)* or purple meadow rue. Fragrant pine needles and aromatic tree fungus are also used.

"These leaves, seeds, and fungi were dried, pulverized, and mixed in the proportions that produce the most pleasing blends and were stored in a decorated buckskin pouch with the other articles of personal grooming.

"A man was expected to be perfectly groomed daily. After his morning dip and bath, he returned to his lodge, ate and dressed in his fine buckskin clothes, combed and oiled his hair, painted his face and applied his perfume, and he was ready for the day.

"A Crow man told me many years ago of his own experience with the use of his sachet when he started his formal education. This man was the pride and joy of his grandparents when he was a little fellow. In fact, as was the custom, the grandparents assumed the responsibility for his training in matters of custom and culture, so he lived with them from the time he was big enough to leave his own parents.

"When he reached school age, he was enrolled to attend one of the reservation day schools. His grandfather was also ready to embark on this new road of adventure. The riding gear for both 'men' was repaired and made ready for that important day and the saddle horses received extra care and attention. Days were marked off the calendar and at night the grandparents prayed over and held their sleeping little fellow tighter to their bosoms and hearts than usual. They knew that they could only prepare the boy for the new life for this was one of the new doors which the white man had opened on their reservation. The boy might just learn the new language to interpret and explain to them the white man's ways and customs.

"In the meantime there was much preparation the grandmother had to make. Extra pairs of moccasins were to be made and put away, so hides had to be tanned and smoked. The boy might happen to find a pool of water to get his moccasins wet in. They would not become stiff as they dried, if they were made from smoked hides. There was much jerky to be made, to roast and pound and mix with just the right amount of wild peppermint to flavor it, and chunks of cooked, hard back, and fat of beef. Some of the dried meat would be roasted and salted for a snack during the afternoon when he played with the other boys. Some days the lunch would be boiled jerky, bacon and a potato, and a piece of buckskin bread baked by the open campfire.

"So as the days came and went, the grandmother would lie awake at night and wonder in her mind what was ahead for their dear little boy who was sleeping so peacefully without a care in the world.

"At last the all-important day arrived! Grandmother was up to greet the new day, build a fire, and start the breakfast. Then it was time for the morning bath. The 'men' were awakened and they both proceeded to the river. The coffee was ready upon their return, so when breakfast was out of the way, the ritual of dressing began. The boy's long hair was combed, oiled, and carefully braided. The red paint was brought out and his face was painted as if he were getting ready for the warpath. New overalls, calico shirt, and new moccasins completed the outfit.

"With their lunch tied on the back of their saddles, the grandfather took a pouch out of his pocket, opened it, and put a handful of sachet contents into his mouth and chewed them thoroughly. He called the boy over and spit what was in his mouth into his hands, after which he plastered the moistened mixture on the little one's head, as well as rubbing some of it on the boy's clothes.

"'Now you are ready for school!' he said and released his grandson to enter the one-room school building.

"The grandfather lingered for several days to make sure his grandson was all right. Each day as the boy came out for recess, the grandfather noticed that the perfume or the sachet that he had previously applied to the boy's head was no longer in his hair. So the grandfather hurriedly chewed up some more and plastered it on the other's hair and sent him back into class. This went on for a couple of days until finally the white teacher appealed to an interpreter to beg 'the old man to quit plastering the boy's hair with *manure!*'

"In time the boy's long braids were cut, his war paint was put away, and he was able to ride to school alone."

SLOUGH GRASS. "This long, tough grass is collected and tied together in a bundle to make a sweat bath switch with. Each person makes and uses his own switch before entering the sweat lodge.

The light switching of the skin is intended to stimulate circulation and more actively increase the elimination of internal poisons through the pores."

SNAKEWEED (*Gutierrezia sarothrae*).   "In Crow we call broom snakeweed *bize:wa:lu:zisse,* which means 'plant the buffalo will not eat.' The leaves and blossoms are harvested, dried, and stored for later use. Uses include: (1) sinus infection; (2) kidney infection; and (3) to reduce swelling. To check these ailments, a strong infusion is made by boiling the leaves and blossoms and straining and re-straining the warm solution. It is sniffed into the nostrils for sinus infection. To reduce swelling, if possible, the area is immersed in the hot solution and soaked and kept hot until relieved or hot compresses are applied. For kidney infection, a milder infusion is prepared as above and is substituted for all liquid intake for the day."

SNAKE WOOD (*Rhus trilobata*).   "The literal translation of the Crow *ia:xasaibale* is 'snake's wood,' meaning a favorite hiding place for snakes. Others call this shrub skunkbush because of its peculiarly foul odor. Uses include: (1) to treat eczema; and (2) to check diarrhea. It should be harvested while the sap is still in the wood. The outer bark is carefully removed and the second layer is scraped off the wood and dried. For eczema, a strong solution is made from the scraped layer of the wood or shrub and used to cleanse and bathe the affected area and let it dry. For diarrhea the same method of preparation is used and the infusion taken after each bowel movement until the condition is relieved."

SNEEZING PLANT (*Helenium microcephalum*).   "The Crow name is *i:wa:pi:axua,* the translation of which is 'what makes one sneeze.' The blossoms are collected after the plant has gone to seed. This is sniffed to induce sneezing to relieve nasal congestion due to a cold. In former days our people also used it to induce sneezing in women who had just delivered themselves of children and were unable to expel the afterbirth. Once the blossoms were held close to their noses and intense sneezing began, the afterbirths usually came out without further delay."

SNOWBERRY (*Symphoricarpos albus*). "*Bizkaxcia* is translated 'dog bush.' The root of this shrub called buckrush or snowberry by botanists is used any time as needed for animals unable to void their own urine. A strong infusion is made from the crushed root boiled in water. A large amount is needed for horses. The solution is strained and poured down the animal's throat. This is repeated until the desired effect is obtained."

SWEETENERS. "When I was young, the Crow knew nothing about white sugar. Our sweeteners came right out of nature—honey (found in hollow tree trunks), box elder sap, cottonwood sap, and honey suckle plant. We were a lot healthier in those times. Diabetes was virtually unknown to us—it was a white man's disease, but something the Crow never got. Indians didn't have the 'sweet tooth' then as they do now. We have paid for adopting the white man's foods and are now atoning for it in sicknesses that our parents and grandparents never had."

SWEET MEDICINE IN THE WATER (*Osmorhiza longistylis*). "The Crow word *bimmu:xba:licikua,* when translated into English, means 'sweet medicine in the water.' Uses include: (1) to treat biliousness from an overactive gall bladder; and (2) to relieve sore throat. This plant is harvested when it is in bloom. The blossoms and the roots are gathered and dried. A tea is brewed from the blossoms and drunk until relief from biliousness occurs. For sore throat, the root is crushed and boiled in water. The tea is used to gargle with. A piece of the root is chewed and the juice swallowed for sore throat."

SWEET SAGE (*Artemisia michauxiana*). "The Crow name is *i:sahcizu:we,* which means 'bunched roots or stems.' Other species such as wormwood (*A. canadensis*) and prairie sagewort (*A. frigida*) are also used. Uses include: (1) incense to purify and deodorize the air; (2) astringent and treatment of eczema; (3) deodorant for the body; (4) foot bath for perspiration; and (5) agent for reviving someone comatose. For incense, dried leaves and fresh leaves and blossoms are sprinkled on live coals in a container and rooms in a house are smudged or in the lodge. For astringent and eczema, a strong infusion is prepared from the leaves boiled in water and strained. This is repeated several times a day to dry up the eczema. The warm tea is patted on and let dry for astringent. A strong solution is prepared as for eczema and patted on the body and let dry for body odor. This is especially effective for underarm perspiration. For a bath to combat foot odor and perspiration, a strong solution is prepared from boiling the leaves and stems. Strain and soak the feet in the solution as hot as can be tolerated. For reviving a comatose patient, the foliage and flowers were burned as incense, the fumes being directed into the nostrils by a paper cone."

WILD PEPPERMINT (*Mentha arvensis*). "Wild peppermint grows in the water along the edge of creeks, ditches, and mountain springs. The Crow Indians call this plant *shu-shu-ah*. Originally it probably meant something else, but according to the language we speak today, it sounds a lot like 'spit, spit.' It could be that the plant has this unusual name due to a very strong mint flavor and you do have to spit after chewing a leaf or two of it.

"To use this plant for tea, pull the plant up by the root, wash and drop the whole plant into boiling water, and set it off the fire to steep until a light green tea is made. Serve hot or iced. The darker the tea, the stronger the mint flavor.

"A year's supply is dried in the sun. The leaves and dried stems are stored in airtight containers and used like Lipton's tea. Our medicine men and women have ground the leaves and stems and boiled them to prevent vomiting. And when boiled with catnip and peppermint and drunk as a tea, it makes a wonderful pneumonia remedy, and can be used to poultice the chest with."

WOLF'S PERFUME (*Artemisia dracunculus*). "False-tarragon sagewort is called *cetizba:ilicitee* by the Crows. It is useful for an eyewash and for snow blindness. A strong infusion is prepared from the stems and leaves. This is strained through cloth or cheese-cloth to remove all of the particles and the solution is dropped in the eyes as needed. For snow blindness, the same preparation is made. The strained leaves are saved and used for a poultice on the eyes and kept saturated with the solution."

YARROW (*Achillea lanulosa*).   "The Crow Indians call it *eih-patci zkizze* or 'prairie dog tail.' It is used: (1) as a poultice; (2) for salves; and (3) for toothache relief. Collect the plant when in bloom. Dry in the sun, pulverize, or break up into small pieces and store in jars or airtight containers. A strong tea to saturate a poultice is made from the boiled plant leaves and used for burns. To make a poultice for boils and open sores, boil the leaves and stems for the poultice. The tea is strained and used to keep poultices saturated. Crushed leaves and stems are boiled with goose grease and strained. Added to congealed fat, this is used for a salve. A strong infusion is made from leaves and stems for toothache and abscessed gums. Hold tea in the mouth as hot as the patient can stand it. Repeat until the aching sub-sides. For abscessed gums, hold tea in the mouth same as for toothache until relieved of pain. Repeat until the swelling goes down."

YELLOW CURRANT BARK (*Ribes aureum*).   "The transla-tion of the Crow *bize:cihtazi'le* is 'yellow gooseberry' or 'yellow cur-rants.' This plant is used in the treatment of canker sores. The inner bark of the stems is scraped and mashed, or if it is dried, it is pulver-ized to powder and applied to the sores in the mouth. Our medicine men and women used to make a poultice of various of the cooked plant parts which was then applied to snakebites. The inner or second bark and stems are used for this purpose. A decoction of this inner bark is also still used for leg swellings sometimes. The fruit is sun dried, stored in buckskin bags, and hung up for winter use. The dried berries are ground, mixed with seed flour, and used to make mush in the morning."

The world of Native American herbal materia medica such as what the late Joy Yellowtail Toineeta represented was once only the medicine of Indians, fur trappers, traders, explorers, and frontiers-men. More civilized whites generally ignored it out of prejudice and arrogance, esteeming it unworthy of their consideration since it belonged to presumed "forest savages." But when the bias finally subsided and doctors and scientists began giving it some serious attention, they happily discovered that the "pharmaceutical spadework" had already been done for them by Native Americans when it came to vitamin C, anesthetics such as cocaine, insulin, antibiotics, and the birth control pill. Without the valuable input of Native Americans, modern medicine would be a great deal poorer; as it is, however, it was greatly enriched by our Indian brothers and sisters everywhere.

Chapter Seven

EARTH MEDICINES OF THE NATIVE AMERICANS

PART III: HEALING CEREMONIES: CHANTING AND SANDPAINTING

(Navajo, Hopi, Pueblo, and Zuni Nations)

The Code Talkers: Wartime Mental Illness
Treated by Healing Ceremonies

The Navajo are the largest Native American tribe in North America and occupy a huge tract of land roughly the size of New England and well over 16 million acres. Their reservation sits primarily in what is known as the "Four Corners" area of the Western United States—the only point in America common to four state boundaries (Utah, Arizona, New Mexico, and Colorado).

Preferring to go by the name of *Diné* (chosen from their own language), which means "the people," they generally despise the more common name given them—*Navajo*—which most of them consider to be just as reprehensible as the *other* "N" word (a vulgar word with racist overtones formerly applied to those of African-American descent).

The Diné (as they shall hereafter be called in the remainder of this text) are a composite group with over 50 separate clans. Formerly they were a predatory tribe who constantly raided the Pueblo and later the Spanish and Mexican settlements of New Mexico, often in alliance with their close kin, the very warlike and once dreaded Apache. But after U.S. Army scout Kit Carson destroyed all their sheep, they meekly submitted to government rule and quit their plundering ways, becoming instead peaceful and law-abiding.

The Diné live in extended kin groups, and traditional inheritance is through the mother's line; women have an important position in the society. Diné religion is elaborate and complex, with many deities, songs, chants, and prayers, and numerous colorful ceremonies, such as the squaw dance and the night chant. The vast mythology includes a creation myth that states that Esdzanadkhi (probably Mother Earth) created humanity.

The tribe has tremendous natural resources, which help to supplement the meager income that members earn from farming and raising sheep. The discovery of oil, gas, and other valuable minerals beneath their land has helped to increase the tribal income, which currently runs close to $20 million per year.

Not too many Americans may be aware of it, but during World War II young Diné men from the reservation were drafted into the Marine Corps and played a crucial part in helping our Armed Forces win the war in the Pacific. At that time our enemies, the Japanese, were breaking American codes as quickly as they could be devised. This placed American servicemen in great peril.

One of the most significant needs in a combat situation of any kind is communications security. This is especially so when troops are spread over a wide area and voice communication is the only certain method of maintaining contact, as it was in the Pacific Theater. This being the case, military commanders and cryptologists had long sought a perfect code, one which could not be broken under any circumstances. Even with the less-sophisticated equipment then in use, it was still possible for Americans to break codes used by the Japanese military, as they, in turn, were able to break ours.

At that time, however, the Navajo language was considered to be one of the world's "hidden languages" in the sense that it had no written form and no alphabet or other symbols. Complicating this situation even more were the facts that, first, the Navajo tongue was confined to the land of the Diné Nation in the American Southwest, and second, there were dialect variations among the clans, and sometimes, within the clans themselves. Finally, only a handful of non-Diné—usually anthropologists or missionaries—could speak this exceedingly difficult language.

During World War I, the U.S. government had attempted using Native American personnel as signalmen, but it was never successful because there were no equivalents for military terms in the Indian languages then being considered. With Navajo, however, it was totally different, and the Diné who were drafted for this unique and peculiar assignment in World War II were able to build a core of words that could effectively serve for military jargon, which would be codes within themselves.

On February 28, 1942, at Camp Elliott, a Marine base slightly north of San Diego, a demonstration was held for the benefit of military brass, which involved five young Diné. This would effectively decide if the Marines were going to draft any Diné young men for a new cryptographic program that the Japanese couldn't decipher. Marine staff officers composed simulated field messages, which were handed to a Diné man, who then translated them into his language and transmitted them to another Diné on the other side of the line. The second Diné translated them into English, in the same form in which they had been originally transmitted. Later, tests in the Pacific under combat conditions proved that classified messages could be translated into Navajo, transmitted, received, and translated back into English much more quickly than messages which were encoded, transmitted, and decoded employing conventional cryptographic facilities and techniques.

This successful demonstration soon led to the U.S. government drafting about 200 young Diné, ranging in ages from 16 (some actually lied about their true age in order to get in) to 25. They would be called "code talkers" and worked exclusively for the Marine Corps in the South Pacific. Eventually an estimated 375 young Diné men became involved in the code talker program.

The first group of recruits devised Navajo words for military terms which were not part of their language: Diné clan names were given to the different Marine Corp units; names of birds (*chicken hawk*) denoted airplanes; the commanding officer was *war chief,* and a major general was *two star.* Alternate terms were provided in the code for letters frequently repeated in the English language. For example, each letter of the alphabet was given three different forms:

ant, ax, and *apple* were the forms of the letter for A. For B, the words were *badger, bear,* and *barrel,* and so on for the rest of the alphabet. To compound the difficulty, all code talkers had to memorize both primary and alternate code terms, for while the basic material was printed for use in training in the United States, the vocabulary lists could not be carried in a combat area for fear of them falling into enemy hands and compromising the whole program.

Once the code talkers completed training at Camp Pendleton near San Diego, California, they were sent to the Pacific for assignment to Marine combat units already deployed. Praise for the success of the program from various Marine divisions in the Pacific Theater poured into the Marine Corps commandant's office almost immediately and continued throughout the remainder of the war. In fact, commanders at all levels heaped endless praise on the program and its participants.

By the end of the war, Diné code talkers had been assigned to all Marine divisions in the Pacific and to Marine Raider and parachute units as well, They took part in every Marine assault, from Guadalcanal in 1942 to Okinawa in 1945. Without their valuable services, it is highly doubtful that America would have won the war in the Pacific.

Unfortunately, a number of years passed before the code talkers finally became recognized in 1969 when the 4th Marine Division Association held its reunion in Chicago. At that time, a group of code talkers was invited to the reunion and presented with a medallion specially minted in commemoration of their services. And further recognition of their dedicated service to the nation in World War II came in December 1971 when the President of the United States awarded a Certificate of Appreciation to each of the remaining survivors.

Those who were recruited for this historical assignment had never seen actual combat. And the extreme violence which war itself always engenders, in which humans are taught to kill other human beings, is something that was totally foreign to Diné culture and religion. While their midnineteenth-century ancestors may have been in the mood for plundering and pillaging innocent victims, these young men were of an entirely different frame of mind. Many of the survivors, in fact, with whom I spoke around the reservation some years ago admitted to being scared out of their wits by the prospects of either being killed or having to kill someone else in order to save their own lives.

Another factor contributed to the fear of many of these young recruits that isn't too well known. Early on in the code talkers program, Marine commanders were worried that the Oriental-looking Diné might be accidentally mistaken for Japanese enemy soldiers. Enlisted Diné were always living in constant fear of this as the following example suggests. Toward the end of the Guadalcanal campaign, an army unit picked up a code talker and sent a message to his Marine command advising that it had just captured "a dirty Jap in Marine combat fatigues and wearing Marine dog tags." A Marine officer immediately hurried off to see if the prisoner was, indeed, an enemy soldier. Imagine his astonishment upon finding one of the young Diné code talkers, sitting dejectedly on the ground with his hands tied behind his back and a GI standing guard over him. The presumed "prisoner" was immediately released into the officer's care, but not before suffering a great deal of fear and humiliation in the process.

Some of the code talker survivors shared with me their own horrors encountered during this period of their lives. Dan Akee of the Kin Yaa'aanii Clan and with the 4th Marine Division saw translation activity at Kwajalein, Saipan, Tinian, and Iwo Jima. "The war was very sad for us. I personally saw dead Marines on the beach at Iwo Jima. It was ghastly. We had to go through many dead bodies, stepping over or trying to walk around the corpses."

Lewis F. Ayze, on the other hand, didn't care to talk about any aspect of his wartime experiences as a code talker. He belongs to the Tachii'nii and Todich'ii'nii Clans and served with the 3rd Marine Division, seeing action in Hawaii, Saipan, and Guam. "These stories I don't care to relate. They are too horrible to repeat. I still suffer a little from their effects after all these years, but some of our tribal medicine men have helped me to cope with them a lot better than I used to."

Fleming D. Begay, Sr., of the Todich'ii'nii Clan, who saw action on Guadalcanal and in Australia, New Zealand, the Gilbert Islands, Tarawa, and the Marshall Islands with the 2nd Marine Division, was "still in my boyhood when all of these events happened. I was eighteen years old at the time. I can't recall [exactly] what I did all those years, but it was quite a *forgettable* experience. I just sort of blocked all of the carnage out of my mind after it was over."

Jimmy Begay of the Naasht'ezhi Diné's Clan and with the 1st and 3rd Marine Divisions at campaigns on Guadalcanal, Taiwan, and Okinawa said: "At Guadalcanal, in August 1942, I was never so scared in my entire life. Even pissed in my pants as I remember. I didn't know if I was going to make it or not. . . . I wasn't at all sure that I was [ever] going to make it [back] to my family hogan."

Lee H. Begay of the Naashgalidine's Clan, accompanied the 2nd Marine Division to Okinawa and Iwo Jima. "I was in combat training in Okinawa. [Those were] rough days [and] rough nights. I was just eighteen at the time, and like so many others from the reservation, young and bewildered by everything we saw and heard and experienced. I believe we lost our native innocence in those places [meaning Okinawa and Iwo Jima]."

Johnny Benally of the Maiideeshgiizhiini and Kin yaa'aanii Clans served with the 1st, 3rd, and 5th Marine Divisions in the Southwest and Central Pacific. His widow recalled her late husband telling her one afternoon, "'Nobody realizes what we had to go through. It was just terrible, absolutely terrible!' My husband never could watch war movies on television after going through what he did over there."

A few code talkers unfortunately had to take human life in order to save their own. Wilsie H. Bitsie of the Bit'aa 'nii and Zuni Tachii'nii Clans was one of these. He was attached to the 1st and 2nd Marine Divisions and saw action, as well as doing code work in the Midway and Aukland Islands, and on Makin, Guam, Emaru, and Wellington. "Why did I kill?" he asked somewhat rhetorically, while staring off into distant space with sort of a glazed look. Then, speaking in slow, halting half-tones, he said, "That whole war has had great psychological bearing on me [ever since], and still does. It robbed me of my youthful innocence and appreciation for life."

Some of the lucky ones, though, believe that they had the protection of the friendly Navajo gods in their favor while seeing action in the Pacific. In fact, those who actively participated in Diné religious rituals before they left and upon returning home again seemed to manage the best from a mental health perspective. Thomas H. Begay of the Tsi'najinii and Ashiihi Clans, who saw action in Hawaii, Enewetak Atoll, Guam, Tinian, Saipan, and Iwo Jima with the 5th Marine Division, was one of those interviewed, who was not only willing but also quite able to discuss his wartime experiences with this author without any apparent reluctance or hesitation.

"We were disciplined. . . . I learned to survive combat. The first hour, I was with my radio, communicating with other floats. I was scared, scared as hell, [with] mortars and artillery shells landing everywhere around me, but I wasn't hit. The Iwo Jima sand was ashy and hard to walk on, but I had to carry my radio and other equipment across it. I was sent to replace Private First Class Paul Kinlacheeny, who was killed on the beach.

"I was awarded six battle stars during my military career for being in major battles from Iwo Jima to the Korean War. I was never wounded or shot but was missed by inches, and missed being captured by only fifteen minutes! I was very lucky, in fact, very blessed to have gotten through that awful time. Maybe because I believe in the traditional Diné ways and felt that the Great Spirit was protecting me. My parents, both very traditional Diné, had ceremonies for me before I left and after I came back. And even while I was gone, they had clothing that I had worn before I entered the service, and used these in some of the ceremonies during my absence. All of these ceremonies protected my physical, mental, emotional, and spiritual well-being, so I could survive and remain fairly normal."

The Healing Chants

Before introducing these particular Native American healing ceremonies, it may be fair to ask if such things really work or just have more of a placebo (imagined) effect. I discovered the truth of this for myself a few years ago when a graduate student in anthropology from the Midwest, contracted my services in the month of December for two weeks to take him to various Native American reservations (Hopi, Navajo, Zuñi, Apache, and Havasupai) located throughout Arizona.

He was overly anxious to meet some "Indian medicine men or shamans" as he called them and prevailed on me often during the initial phase of our extended auto trip as to when we might come into contact with such. Our first stop was in Tuba City at the local high school, where I solicited the help of my friend Howard Begay, a janitor, for translation purposes.

I decided to teach my temporary employer a thing or two about the inherent dangers of excessive zeal. We drove to one man's fairly nice house in town, which had several brand new pickup trucks parked to the side of it. Located nearby was a fancy hogan. I walked up to the Diné fellow to whom such possessions belonged. We shook and then in a very formal way he asked me what my business was.

I informed him that I had it on good authority from my friend Howard Begay, that he was the local "medicine man" for visiting white tourists. He admitted to being such and told me his fee, demanding payment up front. I asked him what one got for $300, and answering with somewhat of a lecherous smirk, he sarcastically replied, "Everything you expect from what the Hollywood Westerns show."

I mentioned to the graduate student that after having endured so much of his pestering, I had finally located an Indian "medicine man" for him. He was thrilled beyond expression and gave me a big hug in front of my interpreter and the other guy, who spoke very good English. He paid the man his price and then proceeded to be methodically fleeced for the next hour with what amounted to nothing but "junk ceremonies." Howard and I remained in our vehicle while this phony shaman serenaded my customer down the primrose path of plain bullsh—. Begay turned to me at one point, inquiring, "Does he know?" I replied, "Not yet, but I'll let him in on our 'little secret' when the guy's finished with him." Begay just shook his head in disappointment and remained silent after that.

A while later, an obviously very happy student came out of the hogan, followed by his trickster, who was now wearing a long war bonnet made from fake feathers that rightfully belonged to the Plains Indians such as the Sioux, but never with the Diné. I thought to myself as I watched the young man finish taking some snapshots of his host, "For a graduate student in anthropology, he sure is kind of uninformed and naive otherwise."

Upon rejoining us inside the car, he was immensely overjoyed and thanked me profusely for this "once-in-a-lifetime experience" (as he put it). I casually asked him as we drove away, what his impressions had been of that visit. He exclaimed with great satisfaction, "Quite frankly, John, this was a lot more than I had expected. I've already gone through two rolls of film and we haven't even fully started our trip as yet." Begay and I looked across at each other in the front seats, but said nothing. We continued to let him rant on for a while about what he imagined to have been a visit with a genuine Diné medicine man.

We drove out of Tuba City a number of miles to a barren section of wasted desert which still legally belongs to the Hopi Nation, but on which, unofficially, several hundred Diné families continue to reside until forcibly removed by the courts. At Begay's signal I turned on to a makeshift trail that wandered off the pavement a ways toward a derelict dwelling. It represented some of the worst poverty to be found on any Native American reservation, but wasn't atypical by any means. The ramshackled unit was a hodgepodge construction of adobe blocks, used lumber, broken windows covered with cardboard, and a roof held in place with tattered tar paper and sheets of rusty aluminum.

The carcasses of several vehicles in different stages of disrepair sat wheelless with their axles resting on cinder blocks. Smoke curled out of an old, dilapidated chimney pipe wired to the back side of the house. The smell of burning cedar wood greeted our nostrils in the crisp winter air. I sent Begay ahead to speak with the occupants inside and make the necessary preparations for our formal introduction, while I casually chatted with the young man.

He asked me why we had come to such an "awful-looking place" as this. To his way of thinking, it was the *last* place someone of his high class and privileged upbringing would have ever thought to come. His had always been a proverbial "silver spoon existence," which is probably why he never batted an eye nor challenged my exorbitant fee of $5,000 for the time involved in pampering this somewhat spoiled son of very wealthy parents.

I had procured some nail clippers from the glove box and was proceeding to give myself a small manicure, when he asked the obvious question I had been waiting for. Without looking up, I replied in demurring fashion, "Isn't this what you paid all those big bucks for? To have me find you some Indian medicine men?"

His eyes got a little bigger and his mouth formed a small "o" of surprise. With this incredulous look plastered on his countenance, he managed to softly croak out, "Then . . . what was *that* back there in Tuba City?" I continued clipping my nails to enhance the effect I desired to leave upon him, and replied in disinterested fashion, "Oh, *that?* Why, *that* was nothing more than *window dressing,* my young friend."

Looking up, I saw my interpreter standing in the open door of the primitive hut, motioning for us to come in. Having finished my deliberate manicure, I opened the glove box and threw the clippers in, banging the lid shut with a loud slam. "Well, let's go," I chimed enthusiastically. He gave me sort of a nervous look, not quite knowing what to expect next of me. I instructed him to leave his camera behind and follow. On the way inside, he whispered in a disturbed tone, "I *demand* to know just what in the hell *this* is all about?"

To which I flashed back a gaze of anger mixed with a rush of adrenaline and hissed into his left ear: *"This,* kid, is what you've paid me to do. You're about to meet the *genuine article* for a change. Just keep your mouth shut, your eyes wide open, and your ears well tuned. You'll probably learn more from this experience than you ever bargained for. And let *me* do all the talking!"

Inside we found an old couple—she was overweight, sixty-something, and sitting on a couch to the left of the entranceway with springs poking up through the ratty cushions. Her husband, his gnarled fingers poking through finger holes at the ends of his gloves, was attempting to warm his hands over a small, wood-burning heater that roared with delight. Begay motioned for the young man and myself to sit on another couch to the side of the medicine man, while he sat directly across from him in the line of vision.

The old Diné spiritual leader appeared to be somewhere in his seventies, which is pretty ancient as Navajo ages go for the elderly. His wrinkled face bespoke much wisdom without the attitude of knowledge so commonly evidenced in today's liberal thinkers and college intellectuals. His eyes patiently looked both of us over, wondering in their mysterious silence why two white men had come all this way on a bitterly cold December afternoon to visit people as insignificant as he and his wife. Discerning this in his quiet gaze, I asked my friend to explain to him the purpose of our visit.

After listening to the explanation given in his own language, he gave a short grunt before responding. Howard turned to both of us and said that the medicine man had just told him that he wouldn't do a traditional chant or 'sing' just for demonstration purposes alone. For within such a chant were embodied prayers to the Diné gods, which made the entire affair quite sacred and not intended for mere show.

Knowing something of the graduate student's mental history from things he had previously told me in confidence, I instructed Begay to tell the other gentleman that the person beside me suffered from a form of mental illness, and that a 'sing' of some sort would greatly benefit his agitated mind.

The graduate student, of course, took exception to what I had just said and began somewhat loudly remonstrating against me. I leaned over and whispered for him to be still, so that the object and purpose in our being there could be fulfilled to his satisfaction. "But I shared that with you in confidence," he whispered back. "I don't care," I responded in low tones. "I'll do whatever it takes to get a 'sing' out of the old man. It just so happens that your condition *is* real and that we've told him *the truth*. Now just sit back, learn, and *enjoy!*"

Begay effectively translated everything I told him to, including the fact that the young man took prescription medication for his mental condition, but that now he was in a state of obvious agitation and needed some vocal therapy to calm him down. The medicine man thought for a minute or so, deciding on what course of action he might take. As he pondered this matter over in his mind, he reached for another piece of split cedar wood, opened the firebox door with his other hand, and threw it inside.

In a few minutes the silence, save for the noise of the crackling fire in the little stove beside the medicine man, was gently broken as he slowly began to "sing" certain memorized lines of a set prayer to his gods. It started out as an almost inaudible drone, then gradually grew in crescendo until it reached medium pitch, where it would see-saw back and forth, sometimes dropping a little in tone while slightly escalating at other times.

The old man's eyes remained closed for the entire time, but his countenance bespoke the absolute sincerity with which he was utter-ing this particular chant. The tonal inflections, the furrowed brow, the serious look, and the occasional slight swaying of his seated body, all indicated the depth of sacredness which he attached to this specific ritual.

Though never understanding one word of what was said, I could tell the gradual effects it was having upon my client as well as myself. He appeared to become very relaxed and in a short while was actually nodding off in an upright position. I, too, became a little bit sleepy, but not as much as he did. When I actually tuned in to portions of this hour-long chant, I discovered that there was a constant repetition of certain sound groups, almost as if the medicine man was repeating certain verses. This impression was only partly correct, I later learned from my friend Begay, who informed me that while the medicine man did repeat *parts* of certain verses often, yet he was always changing other parts of them as he went along so that no two verses ever were exactly alike.

No hypnotist could have ever produced such a depth of sugges-tion or as profound an influence on the mind of another individual, as what this Diné healer had done with my client. Once the ritual was completed, I had to shake the young man to rouse him out of a deep slumber. "Is it over already?" he asked, and then replied in the next breath that the deep effect which it had made inside his head "was as if someone had been massaging my brain for a while."

He was so grateful he wanted to give the old man some money

then and there, but Begay and I quickly interceded and told him to put his wallet away so as not to offend the other person. Begay then asked him in his native tongue what items he and his wife could use the most. The answer came in the form of some canned goods, a sack of beans, a sack of flour, some ground coffee, and a little pouch of loose tobacco. We drove back to Tuba City, where my client purchased these things with his own money. He intended getting double this amount, but again was reminded by Begay and I that to do so would be overpaying, which, in the eyes of the medicine man, would constitute a fraud. We took these goods back to their hovel, where the old, heavyset woman received them with a grunt of thanks, and we departed after that.

The young man was a little disappointed that there was no final hug, handshake, parting words of comfort, or even a managed smile. Begay explained to him that this wasn't the Navajo way at all. That to do so, as the white man does, is thought to bring bad luck. Because then the gods might make the separation permanent, which isn't what any Diné desires to see happen. So they meet and depart without any fanfare as if the get-together was perfectly routine and part of a normal behavioral pattern.

Traditional chants, such as the one performed for the graduate student from Cleveland, are only one aspect of the healing ceremonies of the Diné; the other part is the sandpainting. One usually accompanies the other, but chants may be performed without the latter; however, sandpainting is *always* done in concert with chanting, and never by itself. The husband-wife writing and photographing team of Jake and Susanne Page, who produced the spectacular book *Navajo* (New York: Harry N. Abrams, 1995; p. 118) referred to both of these ceremonies as a form of "cosmic chiropractic," where an individual's psychic spine "is kneaded by story and prayer back into alignment [so that] the balance of things is put right [again]." This is undoubtedly what my client had in mind when he remarked after the chant had ended that it felt "as if someone had been massaging [his] brain for a while."

Most such healing ceremonies usually take place in the evening or in the morning or both, but sometimes necessity may dictate for it

to be done in the afternoon (as was the case with Lowe). The medicine man, more properly called a singer, had to evaluate my client's
psychological condition in his own mind and then decide which of
over 200 different chants would be the most appropriate. These sung
prayers stem from the Diné version of the Creation Story and are of
varying range and complexity but intended for the restoration of harmony. My interpreter Howard Begay later explained to us that the
young man had received a relatively simple one known as the
Hozhoji in Diné or the Blessingway in English.

The old medicine man invoked one of the most powerful Navajo
deities, Changing Woman, who plays a predominant role in Diné religion. This didn't require the elaborate ritual common to most of the
other ceremonies. As its very name implies, it is an act of balance, a
blessing for a person, and it came from Changing Woman, regenera-
tor of life, the everlasting One.

The singer was very careful to make sure that everything was
done in a certain prescribed order and didn't vary one iota from it,
even though he kept changing some of the verses along the way
(which is part of the ritual anyway). It is very important that a singer
perform any ceremony in the same way which he or she had learned it
from former medicine people. The Diné believe that such *exactness* is
critical for the attainment of the harmony desired and the specific
healing sought for.

The chants themselves are handed down from generation to generation; they are all oral, though some of today's modern medicine
men are guilty of laziness and *tape record* all of the known chants
sung by older singers so that they don't have to memorize them. And
when called upon to perform a specific chant, they just fast-forward
their little machines to the one needed in their inventory and play it;
the older singers think this is shameful and not only brings disgrace to
their profession but also offends the Holy Ones (the Diné equivalent
of the gods).

While there are several hundred different songs to be learned by a
prospective medicine man, there are about seventy-two different
ways of praying and none of them are written on any paper or
recorded; these are stored in the mind for future use. Thus, healing

chants are an active and *ongoing* combination of both prayer and song! It takes an average of 25 years to become a proficient singer.

Also, there are different *lengths* of traditional sings: a *short* one usually lasts an hour or so; a *longer* one can run for several hours. While a *small* sing usually lasts an entire evening (5 to 6 hours), a *bigger* sing sometimes can stretch over 5 nights or 10 days!

There was one highly intriguing piece of information that my interpreter friend shared with me in private (for he didn't want Lowe to hear it). Old-time singers such as the one who performed the simple healing ritual for our graduate student are able to put themselves into a partial trance while chanting, which enable them to see ghosts or the spirits of the disembodied that frequently tend to linger around many of us. The prayer and the chanting are like asking these spirits in a nice way to please leave the person alone, and to stay in their own world and let that individual continue with his or her own daily life. Sometimes such malevolent spirits don't want to leave and it becomes more difficult for the singer to persuade them to leave; hence, the mighty exercising of his faith in the Holy Ones in hopes that they will bring their great powers to sway such mischievous spirit entities away for good. The medicine man working on my client's behalf told Begay in Navajo that he saw two powerful spirits hanging around the man while his eyes were shut during the singing and he knew from their appearance that they were troublemakers. Finally, near the end of his chant he saw one of the Holy Ones dressed in *white,* traditional Navajo garb, advancing toward this pair of imps, at which time they grumbled to each other but did depart. That's when he stopped the sing.

The purpose of medicine men and women is to take care of what's wrong *inside* a person's heart, mind, and soul. Regular doctors know a great deal about the human body and how to mend a broken bone, repair a clogged valve, or even treat cancer. But they aren't really trained to deal with the thoughts and feelings of patients—that's where Diné medicine people come in handy.

To understand how such Native American healers work within a culture like the Navajo, you have to understand something about the people themselves. Two salient qualities of the Diné are dignity and happiness. Both spring from their vital traditional faith—faith in nature, faith in themselves as a part of nature, faith in their place in the universe, deep-rooted faith born of their Oriental origin, molded and strengthened by the love in which they live.

There is fine quality in the Diné people—it is evident in their quiet direct manner, their action, their manual dexterity and skill. They bring to their everyday living dignity, vitality, realism, and acceptance of things as they are. Conforming to the pattern of their tradition, they are nonetheless individualists. They have character, they have the ordinary run of human weaknesses, they have humor and a sense of fun, they have their own code of honor. They are also very tenacious. They can be practical to a high degree and are quite poetical.

They are capable of long hours of hard work, and they are just as equally capable of inactivity. There are many good Diné who are strong and dependable, but also a growing number of bad people, who are untrustworthy and weak.

Their powers of observation are photographic. They are immeasurably adaptable to *any* situation that may face them, irrespective of how hard or onerous it may prove to be. They can be exceedingly shrewd, are rather inscrutable and hard to comprehend, and highly intuitive. Among themselves they are a very gentle people as a rule. Through all their unique culture runs a vein of kindness, inherent good manners, and a special quality for which it is difficult to find the right word in English. Perhaps, "integrated personality" is the right attribute I'm looking for, because there is truly a "oneness" about these people in just about everything they do. Simply and quietly they abide by their traditions.

Therefore, it is these very characteristics and virtues of goodness which go into the prayers and songs they offer up. It is, in fact, not only the singer himself (while there are medicine women, *none* are singers) whose traits come through in a healing ritual, but also the very society of which he is a part of. Thus, the singleness of *one* and the totality of *all* are brought to bear during such sacred performances. It is that *combined* energy of self and group which can then inspire wellness in another on all planes: physical, mental, emotional, and spiritual. If "it takes a village to raise a child" (as the well-known title of the popular book by Hillary Rodham Clinton goes), then it *definitely* takes the behavior of a clan *and* tribe to evoke wonderful balance in the healing process.

The Diné have songs of many kinds to fit just about every occasion necessary. There are sacred songs, the chants from the many ceremonies, several hundred as has been previously mentioned. There are songs for an individual and songs for a chorus. A medicine man must know all the chants in every ceremony he conducts. There are songs related to all forms of living creatures, songs of protection, songs to ward off evil. There are songs for daily activities and songs of sorrow, of gladness, and supplication. There are songs about holy mountains and sacred places, just as there are other songs for games and pleasure.

A Diné feels rich according to how many songs he or she has committed to memory. Navajo silversmiths are renowned worldwide for their expert metallurgical craftsmanship. There is great skill in using the hammer correctly, striking blows with the edge of it and producing blows of even strength. Silversmiths like to sing as they work in order to obtain a rhythm of song and stroke so everything is done correctly and turns out nice. A Diné woman sitting outside her hogan by her loom weaving a wool rug of traditional patterns will quietly sing to herself to ensure that her efforts are uniform so that the final design and product turn out perfect.

There are songs for smaller ceremonies, songs for the blessing of a new hogan, a song for the building of a baby's cradleboard, and even songs for the general protection and overall happiness of growing children.

The Diné, probably more than any other people on earth (save for those of African descent), have truly perfected the act of singing, so that it has become for them both an act of consciousness change as well as unconscious routine. One thing I noticed early on in my anthropological studies of the Diné is that they do *not* get depressed like white people and others do. They have learned that song is a potent tool for working with themselves and others though musical sound.

When they sing, they are tuning themselves as instruments to a higher energy field, as we ought to be doing to ourselves more often. They attune the frequencies of their own bodies through the sounds they make in much the same way that musicians will tune the strings of their instruments. But for the Diné it is an *un*conscious effort, while with the latter it is always purposeful and thought out (no musician worth his salt will tune a stringed instrument without paying conscious heed to how it sounds).

This view of the human body as an instrument is a useful metaphor for discussing tuning the body and appreciating it as both a receiver and a sender of sound/energy. To tune, as one would tune a cello, requires that one view the body as a field of frequencies in different vibrational patterns. For instance, frequency of elbow, frequency of earlobe, of knee, of hand, and so forth. Every form in the universe has its own distinct sound and vibration pattern, which is a central belief to the Diné healing ceremonies. When a Diné medicine man employs his voice to tune the body of a sick patient, he may not be able to "hear" the sound patterns specific to the parts of the body intended, but he is trained and disciplined enough to *feel* or, in some cases, to actually *see* them. By these means he is able to know when a pattern is resonating in harmony with the rest of the body field.

When a patient has been tuned and resonates clearly, he or she feels spacious, at ease, in one piece *and* at Peace! In the presence of such a one who is truly at one with himself or herself, others may also feel more relaxed, more spacious and centered themselves.

The operative principle here is the physical law that says a strong vibration will draw weaker, more chaotic ones into its field, and they will correct to its stronger pulse. The person who is strongly centered will also, like a well-tuned instrument, react with sympathetic resonance to the note you sound, allowing your particular vibration to find center, without being drawn away from its own essential tuning. When one centers and strengthens one's own vibrational patterns, one can draw strength and sustenance from the life system of which we are all a part. None of us is ever alone, but we tend to cut ourselves off from the source of our own energies (like so much radio static) when we don't permit inspiration, quite literally sound *inflow*, from the vibrational energies of the rest of creation.

One of the simple, elegant virtues of the act of singing is that it works with inspiration—the flow of melodic sound is the flow of the life force itself. Singing is like recharging our batteries. In song we can connect to deep levels of feeling and energy that are often difficult to reach from everyday consciousness. The Diné learned to do this a long time ago, which explains why they are such a happy and contented people.

Health-Restoring Sandpaintings

The Diné word for sandpainting ('*iikááh*') means "place where the gods come and go." Sandpaintings serve as impermanent altars where ritual actions can take place. But they are much more than that. In their proper setting, if ritual rules are followed, they are the exact pictorial representation of supernaturals. These stylized designs are full of sacred symbols and through consecration are impregnated with supernatural power, thereby becoming the temporary resting place of holiness.

They are essential parts of curing ceremonies and may be performed by medicine men or singers (*hataatsi*) with considerable skill and experience; there are singers, however, who choose only to conduct chanting ceremonies devoid of the sandpainting side (as was the treatment, cited earlier, offered to the graduate student). The chief purpose of sacred sandpaintings is to attract the Holy People so that they will help with the complex curing process. The supernatural power that sandpaintings are believed to contain is dangerous. Which suggests that they can be safely used only in the proper controlled context, at the right time, under the direction of highly trained specialists. They are not "art" in the Western sense of the term for they are not spontaneous creations; rather, the stylized designs created during the ceremonies are strictly prescribed and they are always destroyed at the end of the ritual.

As one (since deceased) medicine man explained to me some years ago, the real purpose of a sacred sandpainting, as well as much of the rest of a healing ceremony, is to bring the timeless people (the

Holy People) together with the people of time (the Earth-Surface People). A sandpainting of this type, carefully done with much prayerful thought, serves as a sort of "cosmic bridge" over which the souls of both parties—supernatural beings and mortals—can cross in order to meet each other at some halfway point on the very edge of time itself.

The religious tradition of sandpainting goes back a number of centuries, but none of the Diné medicine men I interviewed seemed to know just how long this was. It is a generally accepted fact among them that their ancient ancestors borrowed the idea of drypainting, along with other aspects of their unique ritual paraphernalia and mythology, from Puebloan peoples, and then elaborated on it to fit into their own religious system. Some archaeological evidence exists in the form of rock murals at ancient pueblos of Awatovi (Antelope Mesa, Hopi Reservation); Kawaika-a on the Jeddito Wash, Arizona; and Kuaua, a Pueblo IV village on the northern Rio Grande, that have definite stylistic similarities with the Navajo in them.

Some scholars have suggested that Navajo drypaintings were inspired by the impermanent and permanent kiva paintings and altar reredos of the Hopi. The Diné, lacking wall surfaces suitable for permanent paintings as a result of their migratory lifestyle, turned to the use of an impermanent floor medium. But since the Pueblos already used sand and cornmeal paintings which the Navajo could easily see, direct borrowing is just as likely.

Because of their stylistic similarity to kiva murals and the use of designs in rock art, it has also been suggested that Diné sandpaintings originally were permanent, implying that the Navajo rule for impermanency is more of a recent development. The evolution of this rule, therefore, could be a result of the period when the Diné were harassed by other Southwest Indian tribes, by the Spaniards, and later by Anglo-American pioneers pushing westward. Navajos probably began memorizing the paintings for safety, for in this way no one could steal the paintings' power. Indirect evidence for the beginning of this shift, consisting of burned hogans and the building of defensive sites, begins in the early eighteenth century.

The Diné theory of the origin of sandpaintings and the development of rules surrounding their use differs from the customary Anglo archaeological and ethnohistorical interpretation. The Diné believe that sandpaintings were given by the supernaturals to the protagonist of each chant myth, who in turn taught it to the Earth-Surface People. For example:

> Rainboy in the Land-Beyond-the-Sky was instructed for the Hail Chant: "You will not make the paintings in this form in the future. Instead you will use powdered rock—dark, blue, yellow, white, pink, brown, and red. If we give you the paintings on the stuff we use, they will wear out, so it is better to make them of sand each time anew."

Sandpaintings are then a gift of the timeless people. The materials come from evil beings who have been brought under supernatural control.

According to many myths, sandpaintings were originally made on buckskin, unwounded deerskin, cotton, black or white clouds, sky, or spiderwebs. The Franciscan missionaries who roamed the Southwest in the seventeenth and eighteenth centuries found that generally the original paintings were held to be a kind of "sewing" (*naskhá*) composed of five kinds of materials. These were unrolled for the prototype ceremony held in the myth for the protagonist after which they were rolled up and carried home by the deities.

But because of the delicacy, value, and sacredness of the sewings, the gods decreed that sandpaintings would be used by Earth-Surface People. Other reasons listed in the myths include that the "sewings" might be stolen, soiled, damaged, lost, or quarreled over. Also paintings might become material possessions that outsiders would be able to steal. Mythological rationales and supernatural proscriptions mandated keeping sandpaintings impermanent. To disobey would bring disaster, blindness, illness, or death to the individual and drought to the tribe.

Sandpaintings are used in most Diné rites, but are best known in song ceremonials, which are rituals in which a rattle is used, accompanied by singing. Song ceremonials include Blessingway rites, which may or may not have sandpaintings attached with them. Longer Blessingway ceremonies, however, do utilize sandpaintings, but those that are made correspond more to Puebloan cornmeal paintings consisting of small, simple but colorful designs made in vegetal materials as well as pulverized minerals. Extended curing ceremonials include Lifeway ceremonies, performed following an accident, Evilway chants that deal with improper contact with ghosts or witches and aims for the expulsion of evil (though Blessingway is capable of that too), and Holyway chants that correct problems resulting from improper contact with supernatural forces and excess, while protecting against future misfortune. While Holyway chants all utilize sandpaintings, Lifeway chants do not and Evilway chants only rarely do.

A curing ceremony is sponsored by the patient and his or her kinsmen. Their help involves securing the services of the singer, paying his "fee," securing gifts for his assistants, and feeding all who attend the ceremony. For larger chants, this may run to a thousand or more people and expenses are great. Depending on the type of ceremony, expenses vary from twenty-five dollars to several thousand. A ceremony must be held in a hogan, usually in the home of the patient or at that of a close matrilineal kinsman. Because of the time and expense involved, a ceremony is never undertaken lightly. Variation which occurs in a ceremony is due partly to the economic constraints and the ability of the family, the desires of the patient and sponsors, as well as the nature of the specific illness.

Variation can be expected in the performance of chants, because rituals are not permanently recorded and are sporadically performed; there is no organized priesthood and the distances between settlements on the reservation are great. This variation is enhanced by the Diné belief that it is dangerous for a practitioner to teach everything he knows to his pupil and by the need to avoid wearing out sandpaintings and other paraphernalia by constant repetition and use. No singer ever gives two identical performances. Even with this caveat, similarity and stability in ceremonies as well as sandpaintings appear to be remarkable.

Curing works by ritually attacking evil and forcing it under control, hence yielding to good. The ritualistic process may be likened to a spiritual osmosis in which the evil in man and the good of deity penetrate the ceremonial membrane (the sandpainting) in both directions, the former being neutralized by the latter, but only if the exact conditions for the interpenetration are fulfilled. One condition is cleanliness and the ejection of evil so that the place it occupied may be attractive to good powers. The chanter's ultimate goal is to identify the patient with the supernaturals being invoked. He must become one with them by absorption, imitation, transformation, substitution, recapitulation, repetition, commemoration, and concentration.

The purpose of sandpaintings is to permit the patient to absorb the powers depicted. This is done first by sitting on them, next by application of parts of deity to corresponding parts of the patient—foot to foot, knees to knees, hands to hands, head to head. In some chants, parts of the drypainting may be slept on to give more time for absorption; sleep seems to aid the process.

The chanter applies the bundle items to the body parts of the gods, then touches parts of the patient's body with his own—foot to foot, hand to hand, shoulder to shoulder in the ceremonial order—and finally with the bundle equipment. This is an elaborate rite of identification. The powers, represented by the sandpainting, are conveyed indirectly by the chanter through the bundle equipment and his own body to the patient's, all because the chanter has obtained power to do this by his knowledge.

A sacred sandpainting can, therefore, be viewed as the "ceremonial membrane" that allows such a transference to happen. Called irresistibly by their likenesses, the supernaturals impregnate the painting with their power and strength, curing in exchange for the offerings of the patient and singer. The rule of reciprocity governs this exchange.

While most sandpainting compositions are highly complex, even the portrayal of a single figure of the main theme is enough to call the supernaturals to the hogan. This single figure fulfills the functions of the sandpainting ceremony, which are therapeutic, invocatory, commemorative, and above all, highly symbolic.

At the commencement of a sandpainting ceremony, a sandpainting setup is erected in front of the hogan door, while the hogan is cleaned and the central fire moved to one side. Next, the floor is covered with clean, riverbed sand and smoothed with a weaving batten. Colored pigments, which have been collected by the family sponsoring the ceremonial and previously ground with a mortar and pestle on the northwest side of the hogan, are placed in various containers near the central area. These colored pigments (which include sandstones, mudstones, charcoal from hard oak, cornmeal, powdered flower petals, and plant pollens) are trickled through the thumb and flexed forefinger. No adhesive is used because the painting will be destroyed at the end of the ceremony. Although paintings vary in size from a foot in diameter to more than twelve feet square, most are approximately six by six feet, or the floor area of the average hogan.

The average size sandpainting requires the labor of three to six men and takes roughly four hours to complete. The more elaborate the composition, the more time it takes, with the most complex requiring as many as forty painters each working ten hours. Smaller, simpler paintings work, but because power is increased by repetition, larger ones are more effective and, therefore, more desirable. The factors determining size include the amount sponsoring families can afford to spend, the number of available men to make the painting, and finally, the chant in which the painting is used.

Sandpaintings are made freehand, except for the occasional use of a taut string to make guidelines straight and ensure that the main figures will be the same size. Extreme coordination and speed are necessary to make a thin, even line. Mistakes will be covered over with clean background sand and the figure begun again. Anyone may criticize in the quest for an error-free ceremony. Unknown mistakes that could be harmful to the makers or invalidate the ceremony are neutralized by a covering prayer from Blessingway.

Construction, placement of figures, composition, and the use of the ritualized artistic designs are strictly prescribed by the timeless people or Holy People. These rules must be followed exactly in order for the cure to be effective. The same is true for the construction of each figure: when a picture of a Holy Person is made, the entire torso is made first in one color. Then the figure is clothed in a technique called overpainting. Only then is decoration (i.e. masks, headdresses) added. Also, the picture is begun at the center and constructed outward in a sun-wise direction (east to south to west to north). All workers then proceed together following this pattern. Finally the guardian and the paired guardians at the east will be constructed last. The only allowable individual deviations are the kilt designs and the decoration of the pouch which hangs from the waist of many figures.

Subject matter consists of symbolic representations of powerful supernaturals who are invoked to cure the patient. These may be the etiological factors (for like can cure like), human-like portrayals of the protagonist of the myth, figures of Holy People, *yeis* (a special class of timeless people), or various personified beings whom the protagonist met on his or her mythological travels.

Holy People, the most common forms, are depicted as personified plants, animals, anthropomorphic beings, natural or celestial phenomena, mythological creatures, or natural objects, in addition to readily identifiable deities. Animals and plants are also painted in a naturalistic or semistylized form as subsidiary symbols. Location and other important symbols are also shown. While many paintings are illustrations of events occurring in the origin myths, few are actually narrative or realistic.

When the painting is completed, the singer inspects it once more. If satisfied there are no errors, he places the sandpainting setup around the painting, intones a protecting prayer, and sprinkles the composition with sacred pollen (which becomes powerful medicine) in the specific order of construction, ending with the guardian. The painting is now used immediately.

The patient, generally not present during the construction of the sandpainting, now enters and reconsecrates the painting. He sits on a specified portion facing east. The singer, while praying and singing, applies sand from the figures depicted in the painting to matching parts of the patient's body, usually from feet to head, right to left. This procedure is repeated four times along with other ritualistic acts.

These procedures have been said to identify the patient with the deities represented in the paintings. Their supernatural strength and goodness are transferred from the sand via the singer, to the patient.

The patient becomes like the Holy People for he has been able to partake of the nature of divinity. As a result, the patient is dangerous to himself and to anyone who is not similarly immune to so much supernatural power. Violations of ceremonial requirements may reinfect the patient or injure anyone who uses his utensils. For these reasons there are restrictions on the patient's behavior for the four days following the ceremony.

Upon completion of the sand application, the patient leaves, and friends may hastily apply some of the sand to their own bodies. At one time people also collected the corn pollen and some of the sand for later use, but now this practice is extremely rare. As the women leave—for it is presumed dangerous for them to see the erasure—the singer erases the painting in the opposite order in which the figures are laid down. The sand is deposited north of the hogan under a lightning-struck tree. Material from each sandpainting forms a separate pile usually placed just north of that deposited on the previous day. Some think that the disposed sand acts as a barrier to the return of evil spirits which have been driven to their home in the north.

As a sacred object containing what is sincerely believed to be very dangerous power, a sandpainting, like masks or medicine bundles, should be used with respect at all times. It is feared as well as revered. The painting never remains in a pristine form unattended, for the longer it remains intact, the greater is the possibility that someone will make a mistake in its presence and cause harm. Therefore, sandpaintings should never be made in a permanent form, medicine men insist. They think that a layman who made one, especially outside the controllable environment of the ceremonial, and did not have the necessary knowledge and hence power, would be harmed. The paintings would draw the Holy People who, because of the principle of reciprocity, would have to come. But they would be highly displeased because their rules had been disobeyed and they would bring sickness and possibly death to the offender.

Given their sacred nature, it is not surprising that making sandpaintings in a permanent form and using them for commercial purposes was unpopular. Use in any secular context was in direct opposition to rules governing Diné religious practices and was interpreted as an affront to deeply held beliefs. Most Navajos were and still are afraid to disobey the Holy People and will not reproduce sandpaintings in any permanent form, particularly those which strive to be exact replicas of ceremonial designs.

But given the changing nature of all cultures, it is not uncommon to find Diné sandpaintings being made now as permanent, secular items; they have been used for a variety of mundane purposes. Beginning in the latter part of the nineteenth century, sandpaintings were reproduced outside their ceremonial context. Anthropologists used them to illustrate books and articles on Diné religion. Navajo weavers incorporated the design motifs in rugs. Designers used them to decorate public buildings, fabric, and dishes. And finally, Navajo artists used them as decoratives and fine art. By 1920 some types of sandpaintings had shifted to the realm of everyday life. The function of sandpaintings became multiple. This included education, decorative art, historic documentation, aesthetic pleasure, economics, and the prevention of culture loss in addition to their religious functions.

The development of secular sandpaintings, however, from sacred ones was often a painful and arduous process. It involved technological innovations, marketing developments, education of potential consumers, increased contact between Diné and Anglo-American cultures, and last but by no means least, cultural and ideological changes by Diné artists and singers. This process is not yet completed; as happens when new norms which test beliefs are developed, conflict ensued among the Navajo and disagreement over the boundaries of the new concept of secular and commercial sandpaintings persist.

Nearly all commercial sandpainters contend that as a distinct class of objects, the items they produce are not the same as sacred paintings and that they are, therefore, safe to make. A few sandpainters, however, have maintained that commercial sandpaintings are not mundane but are living entities just like their sacred counterparts. These painters are blurring the line that others are trying to draw between sacred and commercial sandpaintings. They protect themselves by saying a prayer upon starting and completing each painting. This blesses the painting, making it a semisacred object, and at the same time it informs the Holy People that their likenesses have been drawn not out of disrespect but to bring blessings to the owner and maker.

One painter reported sprinkling cornmeal on the commercial paintings each morning, talking to the deities so that they would understand and approve, stressing that he was making the paintings correctly as taught by the forefathers. By and large, however, commercial sandpainters use artistic devices and methods analogous to those developed by singers at the turn of the century as the means to separate the two types of sandpaintings.

Besides the obvious religious symbolism involved, color is really at the heart of Diné sandpaintings. Colors are chosen with deliberate care in order to invoke the most potent healing medicine possible. This principle is really no different in the white man's world. I spoke by telephone with Eric Johnson, head of research for the Chicago-based Institute for Color Research in the beginning of 1999. This place collects scientific information about the human response to color.

He noted that a customer spends only the briefest amount of time at the supermarket deciding which products and which brands to buy, and the colors food manufacturers use to package their products are chosen with a great deal of forethought and advance planning in order to sway consumers in what are sometimes split-second buying decisions.

But color isn't all that's used to influence you at what marketers call the "point of purchase," he observed. The shape of a food package is meant to entice, too, as are (of course) various price promotions. But above anything else, he stated, "Color works the strongest marketing magic of all, and marketers know it and take full advantage of this understanding." For example, there has been "a long-standing tradition in the packaging industry that if you want a product to sell *really well,* put it in red and white. Campbell's soup, Carnation Instant Breakfast, and Marlboro cigarettes come to mind, as a few of the top sales leaders in their respective fields because of their distinctive-looking red-and-white packaging.

"Red stimulates feelings of arousal and appetite," Johnson told me. He explained that when the eye sees red, the pituitary gland sends out signals that make the heart beat faster, the blood pressure increase, and the muscles tense—all physiologic changes that can lead to the consummation of a purchase. (No wonder so many foods have red somewhere on their packaging.)

Red is also considered a "warm and inviting color," he mentioned. You'll frequently see at least some red on boxes of pasta, he commented. It evokes shared, hearty Italian meals.

Just look at the influence that green has today, he continued. "Thirty years ago, it was barf color. But then it became associated with the environment, and that meant prohealth. It has morphed 180 degrees." Just how much green's reputation has come around has been underscored in a recent study conducted by the University of Illinois Food & Brand Lab, which examines how consumers make purchasing decisions at the point of sale. A covert color switch was made on a popular sweet treat. O'Henry candy bars, normally found in yellow wrappers, were put in green ones instead. When the bars were seen in green, consumers said they had fewer calories, more protein, and fewer calories from fat than when they were in their usual packaging.

Green's astonishing effect is probably why Hershey's reduced-fat Sweet Escapes candy bars have green on their wrappers, just as Healthy Choice frozen dinners are packaged in largely green boxes. Decaffeinated coffee tends to come wrapped in green, too, while regular coffee often comes in "robust" red.

By itself, white suggests reduced calories. Sales of sugar-free Canada Dry Ginger Ale increased when its labels incorporated more white, Johnson noted. Silver also means fewer calories. A bottle of Diet Coke is mostly silver; a bottle of regular Coke, mostly red. Get it?

Yellow is the fastest color that the brain processes, he explained. Thus, he said, it's a real "attention getter for sure." There's also "a mythic thing about yellow being a happy color," he added. For those reasons, it's not surprising that yellow is a very common color in supermarkets, appearing on everything from boxes of Cheerios to Domino Sugar to Triscuit wafers to Hellmann's mayonnaise.

In sociologic studies, Mr. Johnson told me, orange indicates affordability. It suggests, "I'm easy, I'm cheap," perhaps because it's not considered a classy color. But its suggestion of accessibility and affordability make it a good color for such "everyman" products as Arm & Hammer Baking Soda, Burger King meals, and Stouffer's frozen entrées.

Rich browns indicate "roasted" or "baked," the Institute for Color Research's department head pointed out. This is most likely why you'll often see brown as a background color on things like bags and boxes of gravy and cake mixes. Brown also suggests rich flavor—a reason it often appears on cans of coffee.

The only color you won't find much of on food packages is blue. People generally want the colors on their boxes, bottles, and cans to reflect what's inside. Mr. Johnson put it this way to me: "Human beings require congruency of color in order to buy the goods. People just won't buy baked beans in a purple can, no matter how good they may taste or how inexpensively priced they are. Beans aren't purple!"

The same type of careful planning and color coordination are widely utilized by Navajo sandpainters but obviously for very different reasons—in their case it is with the view to bring about a healing when sacred sandpaintings are temporarily created, or to present something with greater permanency that is aesthetically pleasing to the eye of those purchasing commercial sandpaintings. The latter, in fact, have become much more colorful than the former through the inclusion of new and vivid colors.

Navajos recognize five predominant colors in sacred sandpaintings: white, black, gold, blue-gray, and red-brown. Brown, pink, and variegated colors occur less frequently. All colors are solid and dominant, and there is no shading. While these colors are still common in commercial sandpaintings, bright turquoise blue, green, bright red, shades of brown, tan, and beige are regularly added to the painter's palette. Painters are increasingly distinguishing shades in sandstones and giving them distinct names. Gray is rarely used in sacred sandpaintings because it is associated with monsters and symbolizes evil, dirt, indefiniteness, and fear, but is found in commercial sandpaintings. Thus it appears that the colors are losing or have lost some of their symbolic significance.

It is clearly evident that Diné medicine men practice a form of color therapy without really knowing it. The greatest focus of concentration is always on the symbols themselves, while the colors comprising each of them often take a back seat in terms of attention importance. Color therapy as practiced in the white man's world is a form of energy healing in much the same way that sacred sandpaintings are with the Navajo.

It isn't totally understood as yet just how color therapy works, but there are four theories. Some researchers claim that colored lights promote the binding of neurotransmitters to receptors, which combats depression. The second theory is that the wavelengths of colors alter brain waves, permitting patients to access subconscious emotions that may be at the root of an illness. The third theory is based on the traditional Chinese medicine belief that disease is caused by an excess or deficiency of *qi* (vital energy or life energy) in a particular organ. Different colors are thought to restore the balance of that energy. The fourth theory claims that color wavelengths travel along the optic nerve and enter the brain's pituitary gland. The pituitary gland signals other endocrine glands to secrete hormones that either excite or calm the body.

There are a small handful of recent studies that have documented the benefits of directed colored light. One, which was published in *Biology of the Neonatre* in 1997, reported that within three hours blue-light phototherapy eliminated the yellow coloring caused by infant jaundice in 5 of the 10 babies studied. The other five infants experienced moderate relief with green-light phototherapy.

Another study, published in the *American Journal of Psychiatry,* compared green light with red light in the treatment of depression associated with seasonal affective disorder (SAD). Two hours of looking at green light over the course of one week reduce depression symptoms in more than half of the 14 patients tested. The same amount of exposure to red light wavelengths had no effect.

Now Diné folk healers are simple folks and use natural elements from the world around them to create simply designed, though highly complex sacred sandpaintings. They aren't into having patients sit in front of a strobe that flashes colored light or having them lie down and letting the colored light be directed at them. Nor do they apply color to acupressure points with different colored hand-held glass rods in a process known as colorpuncture.

They don't need such high-tech gadgets or fancy systems to get color to their patients. They simply have those whom they're treating merely look at the sandpaintings and then immerse themselves in them by sitting down in the center of them. This accomplishes the same effect that the other, more sophisticated (read "*un*natural") technologies purportedly do.

Those desiring to employ *some* form of modest color therapy in their own healing experiences would do well to at least imitate the Navajo *in principle,* though not necessarily executing a sandpainting for themselves. I've taken what is considered by many color therapists to be the best array of colors for healing, daily activity, and emotions. Beside each of them I've given terse descriptions that best fit each one, together with those foods that naturally belong there. If the reader will carefully study the list below and choose those colors (and foods if needed) for a particular situation, then he or she will soon discover what Diné medicine men have known for centuries—that the world of color (as expressed by them in their clever sandpaintings) does indeed make a difference in how one thinks, feels, and behaves!

> FLESH SPECTRUM: Harmony, organization, practicality—
> peach, apricot, tan figs.
> VIOLET SPECTRUM: Culture, idealism, psychic—eggplant,
> beet, Concord grape.
> RED SPECTRUM: Romance, physical life forces, elegance—
> red bell pepper, rhubarb, cherry, currant, cranberry, tomato,
> radish, strawberry, watermelon.
> ORANGE SPECTRUM: Creativity, kindness, joyfulness—or-
> ange, tangerine, mango, cantaloupe, pumpkin, carrot.

YELLOW SPECTRUM: Glorifying God, analytical, cheerfulness—papaya, banana, banana squash, Hubbard squash, corn.

GREEN SPECTRUM: Balance, fairness, peacefulness—cucumber, bell pepper, kiwi, celery, lettuce, broccoli, asparagus, parsley, watercress.

BLUE SPECTRUM: Spiritual, serenity, soulfulness—blueberry, boysenberry, plum, bing cherry, Indian blue corn.

WHITE COLOR: Holiness, purity, illumination—parsnips, rutabaga, cauliflower, onion, Queen Anne cherry, Chinese litchi nuts, pecans.

GRAY COLOR: Neutrality, mutual agreement, subdued tone— Some seaweeds such as kelp, some algaes, some mushrooms.

BLACK COLOR: Consuming emotion, finality, drawing— Blackberry, black raspberry, prunes, raisins, black mission figs.

Each of our senses is attuned to color in some way, whether we are consciously aware of it or not. Certain colors can bring us pleasure and joy, while others may deliver courage and hope. The vibratory nature inherent to all colors of the spectrum are fully penetrating and reach the very depths and centers of our physical, mental, emotional, and spiritual existences in ways we know not of. Viewing the appropriate colors, whether it be in a Navajo sandpainting or something we've created for ourselves from colored paper, will center the body, balance the mind, steady the heart and liver (the seats of emotions), and square the soul with the Great Spirit, the Giver *and* Sustainer of Life itself!

Chapter Eight

HISPANIC AMERICANS AND THEIR FOLK MEDICINE CONTRIBUTIONS

*(Mexico, Cuba, Puerto Rica, Colombia, Peru,
and El Salvador)*

Coming to America

I t started with Christopher Columbus (actually Christobal Colón) in 1492, when he "sailed the ocean blue" and happened to discover the Americas. He and his crew were the first real Hispanic immigrants to the Western Hemisphere and the tide of brown hasn't stopped since.

Daring and ruthless adventurers from Spain known as conquistadors—Francisco Pizarro, conqueror of Peru, and Hernán Cortez, conqueror of Mexico, were the greatest of their kind—virtually annihilated the great Indian civilizations of the New World in the sixteenth century and subjugated the many survivors to a life of slavery. Spanish soldiers frequently intermarried with local Indian populations, resulting in the emergence of new ethnic identities; the best known of these by far was the genetic union between Spaniards and Aztecs in central Mexico, resulting in the Mexican race.

Not all Spaniards were cruel and barbarous, however. With the conquistadors came hundreds of Spanish priests, who established numerous missions throughout Mexico and eventually went up into the American Southwest and California to do the same there. Their purposes were often twofold: One was to obviously try and convert what they presumed to be heathen Indian savages to Christianity, and the second, more nobler effort, was to educate these Native Americans in their ways so as that they could provide better lives for themselves. These mission outposts provided the real backbone for Spanish rule and influence. Many missions were agricultural, growing fruit and cereals, and rearing livestock; the labor force was largely Indian. But there were also Hispanic settlers as well; in 1821, they probably numbered around 5,000.

The United States has always been a nation of immigrants. Over the years more than one hundred ethnic groups have been represented here. But even though the nation has been settled by people from around the world, most Americans can trace their individual origins to Europe somewhere. At the beginning of colonization, the English dominated migration to the New World. Then they were joined by Scotch-Irish, Germans, French Huguenots, and black Africans.

But then new immigration patterns began emerging in the middle-to-late 1850s. Around the time of the Civil War, millions of newcomers again swelled the population. Northern Europeans dominated this wave of immigration as Irish, Germans, Swedes, Danes, and Norwegians came by the tens of thousands. Later, in the years around the turn of the century and before World War I, the origins of newcomers expanded to include people from southern and eastern Europe—Poland, Russia, Italy, Greece, Yugoslavia, and Romania.

Since World War II, immigrants have often been refugees. Since the mid-1970s, immigrants from Spanish-speaking nations—Cuba, Haiti, El Salvador, and most of all Mexico—as well as Asians from Korea, Cambodia, Vietnam, and Thailand have filled the roster of new arrivals.

During the Great Depression minorities suffered more than the general white population. This was especially the case with the Hispanic population. Ever since 1920 they had been moving in huge numbers to Texas, California, and other parts of the Southwest. Mexican-Americans worked most often as farm laborers, an occupation less well protected by federal and state laws than other types of work. When the creation of the dust bowl sent thousands of ruined farmers to California, Mexican-Americans found it harder than ever to make a living. Competition among workers drove some farm wages as low as nine cents an hour. Efforts to unionize were often met with legal action and guns. The CCC (Civilian Conservation Corps) and WPA (Work Projects Administration), both funded by the U.S. federal government, were helpful to some Mexican-Americans, but migrant workers could not qualify if they had no permanent address.

Those fortunate enough to eke out some kind of meager subsistence did so often living in ramshackled quarters at best. The main source of amusement back then was the radio, but there were no Hispanic stations as there are today. Mexican-Americans able to understand sufficient English were entertained by programs geared strictly for white audiences. Those Mexican-Americans lucky enough to own radios were treated to a variety of programming. In the afternoon were serials portraying romantic adventures and small-town life, such as "The Romance of Helen Trent," "Ma Perkins," and "The Guiding Light" (which by the way, happens to be the longest running radio-TV soap opera anywhere in the world). The main characters in these stories were female, but it was difficult for Mexican-American women to readily identify with such fictional persons.

Later in the afternoon, there were adventure stories for children, including "Little Orphan Annie," "The Green Hornet," and "The Lone Ranger." The evening had excellent dramas and variety programs featuring such stars as Bob Hope, Orson Welles, Eddie Cantor, Jack Benny, and George Burns and Gracie Allen. I've listened to some of those old programs and have examined a few of their scripts. It was unfortunate that whenever Mexican-Americans were portrayed in some way in any of these programs, it was invariably always in negative terms. They would either be portrayed as helpless ignoramuses to be rescued from dilemmas of their own making by white people or else be the butt of endless jokes when depicted as lazy and shiftless. In fact, the proverbial long Mexican siesta following an afternoon meal became a trademark for much of the gag material used by comedians then.

For outside entertainment, families usually went to a movie, which back at that time only cost a mere 25 cents for daytime matinees or 50 cents for an evening flick. Stars such as Greta Garbo, Joan

Crawford, Marlene Dietrich, and Loretta Young played in dramas that reflected a life of sophistication and luxury. This was done deliberately because people in pinched economic circumstances got vicarious, or secondhand, pleasure in watching the make-believe frolics on the silver screen. But not so with those Mexican-Americans able to afford such things periodically and who understood enough English to know what was going on in the film. Whenever they saw themselves portrayed, it was always in demeaning ways, being typically in roles of traditional servitude, and sometimes given to speaking with bad accents for comic relief. To add insult to injury, however, their kind were usually played by second-rate *white* actors, who mimicked the parts of ignorant Mexican-Americans pretty well.

Many Mexicans had become American citizens in the mid-1800s when the United States annexed the Southwest following the Mexican-American War. During and after World War I, a large number of Mexicans crossed the border to work in the States. Most of them were either migrant farm laborers in the area's orchards, vegetable farms, and cotton fields or miners and railroad workers. Many came under a legal work contract. But many also crossed the Rio Grande without a passport. But regardless of how they came, Mexican-Americans played a major role in the economic growth of the Southwest.

During World War II, many Mexican-Americans served in the armed forces. When they returned to civilian life, they were determined to do something about the poor conditions under which most of them lived. Known more popularly in those times as Chicanos, they often suffered from discrimination in housing and wages. In addition, many were handicapped by the lack of job skills and the inability to speak English well. They wanted better opportunities to become educated and to earn a living.

Mexican-Americans were shocked into organized action by an insult to the family of Felix Longoria, a Mexican-American war hero killed in the Philippines. The only undertaker in his hometown in Texas refused to let the Longoria family use his funeral home because they were "disgusting wetbacks" (the term this white man actually used in reference to them). The American G.I. Forum was organized to protest this and other injustices to Mexican-American veterans.

Soon after, Ignacio Lopez founded the Unity League in California to register Mexican-Americans voters and to promote candidates who would represent them. The league also succeeded in having segregated classes for Chicano children outlawed in the state. Similar voter registration groups were formed under various names in Arizona and Texas.

Ever since the 1970s, Mexico has led all other Latin American countries in the number of immigrants flooding into the United States. These include both legal and illegal. Though actual statistics are hard to come by, some unofficial reports put the number of Mexicans entering the United States legally and otherwise as high as 1.8 million a year. This tremendous influx from south of the border began to alarm many white middle-to-upper-income conservatives, who feared a "real invasion" of some sort by such foreigners. In the mid-1980s our nation was caught up in hysteria over so many Mexicans streaming northward, into what they saw as "a land of opportunity and plenty" in which to make better lives for themselves and their families.

The country's esteemed lawmakers passed the Immigration Reform and Control Act to try and stop this, or at least slow it down, and at the same time appease voting districts back in their own home states. As things turned out, though, it only hurt immigrants. Employers stopped hiring brown-skinned, brown-eyed, and black-haired people with "foreign-sounding" names, so as not to get in trouble with the immigration laws.

An "ABC News 20/20" special hosted by correspondent John Stossel on December 14, 1990, put the current problems in some perspective. Dr. Rafael Martinez, then the executive director for the North County Chaplaincy in San Diego, California, was one of those interviewed.

STOSSEL (voice-over): Rafael Martinez points out that we give immigrants contradictory messages. We say, "Don't come, it's illegal." But we also say, "We need you to do the work that our own people won't do anymore."

DR. MARTINEZ: Who picks up all those crops and brings them to our table ridiculously cheap? These are the people who do it. . . . [Whites] need these people to come and take care of their landscape, beautiful manicured yards. They need. the women to come and be their maids. Yes, that they want, at a very low price. Yet, they would also like them to just disappear at the end of the day and go off where they can't be seen or bother anyone.

Snippets of interviews with several different Mexican-Americans were included in Stossel's report. Speaking through an interpreter, one immigrant noted: "I think that Americans see us from a racial perspective without taking into account that by being here in their country, we are doing the gringos a big favor, because all of the hard labor is done by the Mexicans, by Latinos, the only ones who aren't afraid to get dirty or do extremely hard, heavy, physical work every day." Another immigrant wondered aloud: "Why are we Mexicans discriminated against so cruelly by Americans when we harvest their crops in their fields, clean their bathrooms in their homes, and mop and scrub everything else in their beautiful houses? *Let's see them do this and like it!*"

Since then, attitudes have changed for the better, and fortunately most of the American public today is far more accepting of Mexican-Americans than they were in the past. The most recent 2000 national survey also shows that within a decade the Hispanic population, at its present growth rate, will overtake and surpass that of Black Americans, making them then the nation's largest minority group.

The Practice of Curanderismo
Along the Texas Rio Grande

A prevailing idea in American culture is that if you really put your mind to something hard enough, there is no obstacle that cannot be overcome nor challenge successfully met. In medical terms, it's conceptualized as being "mind over matter." This, in essence, pretty well summarizes a great deal of the workings of a unique folk medical system common to Mexican-Americans in the American Southwest known in general terms as *curanderismo*.

Within this broad alternative healing system are a variety of folk healers, each using a set of techniques exclusive to their particular specialty; there is always, however, an overlapping of methods and materials among these specialties. These healers include *parteras* (midwives), *yerberos* (herbalists), *sobadores* (people who treat sprains and strained muscles), and the very popular and most plentiful of all, *curanderos* (male healers)/*curanderas* (female healers). While the former groups may use herbs, massage, chiropractic, and even prayers sometimes in their practices, it is the last group who are deemed the most professional at being able to manipulate both the supernatural world as well as the physical one.

All of the data for this chapter was collected by myself from Mexican-American informants (both healers and patients) as well as some orthodox medical doctors (both Hispanic and white) residing in the Lower Rio Grande Valley of southern Texas, which is composed of the Texas counties of Cameron, Hidalgo, and Willacy on the American side, plus the border region of Northern Tamaulipas in northern Mexico.

The Valley, actually a flat area formed by the flood plain of the Rio Grande, has a somewhat unusual habitation pattern on the United States side where the majority of my research was conducted in the mid-1980s. A habitation strip no more than fifteen miles wide at the widest point has been formed by a nearly continuous series of small towns (population 2,000 to 50,000) running from Brownsville at the mouth of the Rio Grande itself to Mission, approximately 65 miles upstream. This strip is bordered by, and often liberally interspersed with, citrus groves and agricultural fields. This makes the entire region an inextricable rural-urban mixture.

Agriculture has always been the main industry. But there is an enormous industrial base on both sides of the border, including a number of recently developed "sister" plants and *maquiladoras* (assembly plants) representing such well-known manufacturing giants as Motorola, Panasonic, GE, Ford, and others. Thus, the area is neither rural nor urban, but a complex mixture of the two.

The 2000 Population Census of the United States estimated that of the roughly three-quarter million people residing in the area, some 83.13 percent are Mexican-Americans, about 16 percent are Anglo-Americans, and the remaining fraction is divided between blacks and Asians. Nearly everyone lives in a basically urban environment, including most of the farmers and farmworkers who work the land.

The American side of the border contains numerous small and medium-sized towns, the largest of which are Brownsville and McAllen. On the Mexican side can be found two major population centers, Matamores and Reynosa, plus scattered ranches and farms. On the Mexican side of the border live nearly one million people. With the exception of the immediately adjacent aforementioned Mexican border cities, the Valley itself is somewhat isolated. The nearest towns of any significant size are Corpus Christi and San Antonio, 130 and 250 miles away respectively.

This relative isolation, along with the extreme ease of movement between the United States and Mexico, causes the Mexican border towns to have both a strong cultural, as well as economic, impact on the entire Valley. Part of the impact comes from the huge population base on the Mexican side of the Rio Grande River. They account for as much as 60 percent of the retail trade in the whole Valley. They also provide a large labor pool that far exceeds the demands and thus keeps wages depressed, plus makes both seasonal and permanent underemployment a chronic problem for Valley residents. The result is that the Lower Rio Grande Valley contains two of the poorest statistical areas surveyed in the last population census.

The demographic characteristics of the Valley are as interesting as its economic characteristics are grim. The population is quite young, over half being under 30 years of age, by current estimates. The area is distinctly bilingual and bicultural. The population dynamics of the Valley are further complicated by the presence of approximately 145,000 migrant farmworkers who make the Valley their home, but who spend from 3 to 6 months out of the area participating in the usual migrant stream northward. Finally, an estimated 250,000 winter residents, most of whom are retired, affluent, and well educated, make the Valley their home between October and March. All of these characteristics combine to make this Valley, in particular, an area of key interest for social scientists conducting anthropological research into folk medicine on the American side of the border.

I spent almost a month in the area, working both sides of the border, but did my principal research on the American side. The information contained here was obtained from 315 informants ranging in age from 15 to 83, but focusing most heavily on the 28-to-57 age range. All of the informants I consulted with identified themselves as Mexican-Americans: 57% of the information was given by individuals born in the United States and 43% of the data was collected from informants born in Mexico. Women usually predominated in my investigative work: 83% of what I gathered came from females, as opposed to just 17% collected from males. (This finding holds true, as a rule, in the whole alternative medicine arena in America, where women tend to be the most active consumers and participants.)

Does Folk Medicine Work?

Scientists who've analyzed a number of the botanicals involved in many Mexican-American home remedies, have discovered that a number of them have valid chemical applications for the problems and conditions for which they're used. But what about nonplant remedies that are more psychological than physical in their makeup? Do they bring healing success in their own way, or are they more fiction than fact? I'll let you be the judge on this one with regard to the following case.

The typical symptoms of systemic lupus erythematosus (SLE) are as numerous as its pharmacologic treatments. Hemolytic anemia, vasculitis, synovitis, lymphadenopathy, nephritis, hepatitis, cerebritis, serositis, and rashes may respond positively to any of the following agents: aspirin, corticosteroids, antimalarial and myelo-suppressive alkylating drugs, not to mention a plethora of synthetic, nonsteroidal, antiinflammatory concoctions. Apparently, though, as the true case below will show, there is another treatment involving folk magic, that while placebo-based, may indeed be of powerful, psychological influence. Or put another way, really a case of "mind over matter" in the fullest sense of the phrase.

While I was doing research on the American side in the Lower Rio Grande Valley of southern Texas in 1985, an American doctor in a local clinic called to my attention the situation of a 32-year-old Mexican-American female and even permitted me to examine her medical records. As I relate her symptoms and condition here, it is necessary that I use the proper medical terminology in the event that some of my readers are trained health professionals and understand the jargon involved. This way they can better appreciate the final outcome which originated with a *curandera* who couldn't spell her name, much less write, but had a solid reputation in the area for her remarkable healing skills. Therefore, I beg the indulgence of lay readers over the next several paragraphs and apologize in advance for using data that may not always be fully comprehended without some sort of medical background.

The female patient involved here, whom I will simply call Luisa, became ill with weakness, hepatomegaly, and intermittent lymphadenopathy. The clinic to which she went documented high ESRs (erythrocyte sedimentation rate or red blood cell sedimentation rate), polyclonal gammopathy, and mild anemia. Also found were RBC (red blood cell) and WBC (white blood cell) casts and a moderate amount of albumin in her urine. Biopsy specimens which my doctor informant obtained from her liver and lymph nodes disclosed nonspecific inflammatory changes. The diagnosis of SLE (systemic lupus erythematosus) was established only when antinuclear antibody and lupus erythematosus clot test results (formerly negative) turned out to be quite positive.

The patient's anti-DNA level was 68 units per deciliter (dL) of blood (normal being 10 units/dL). Her serum creatine level was 0.7 milligrams per deciliter of drawn blood. Shortly after prednisone therapy, 60 milligrams per day, was begun, the hepatomegaly, albuminuria, and lymphadenopathy disappeared, and the patient felt pretty well after that. The steroid dose was tapered. One month later, levothyroxine sodium therapy, 0.20 milligrams per day, was begun because total and free thyroxine levels were found to be too low.

The attending doctor (my informant) diagnosed smoldering lupus nephritis, as indicated by the patient's persistent RBC and WBC casts, and protein in her urine. Whereupon he again prescribed 60 milligrams per day of prednisone, in four divided doses, with tapering off once her sedimentation rates and results of urinalysis had returned to normal.

She became edematous, cushingoid, and intermittently irrational shortly thereafter. So a few months later the same doctor prescribed a mild daily dose of azathioprine to help reduce the dose of prednisone. However, when the woman's serum creatine levels began to rise again, she was given a renal biopsy and high-dose, parenteral pulse steroid therapy (1,000 milligrams of methylprednisolone intramuscularly every three weeks). The biopsy revealed membranous and focal glomerulonephritis and immune complex disease.

When high-dose, sustained prednisone (60 milligrams per day) and cyclophosphamide were recommended, the patient instead insisted on visiting a local *curandera* in the area, known widely for her recognized folk-healing skills. The day she left the clinic, her blood test results disclosed the following values: hemoglobin, 9.0 gs/dL; serum creatine, 1.5 mg/dL; serum complement (C3), 63 mg/dL (normal being 70 to 176 mg/dL); C4, 36 mg/dL (normal being 16 to 45 mg/dL); and ESR, 149 millimeter per hour. A urinalysis done prior to the patient's departure disclosed proteinura (4+), WBC and RBC casts, and a trace of glucose.

Imagine the surprise of distraught family members and her astonished but somewhat skeptical clinic physician, when the patient returned three weeks later without any of the typical signs for SLE. She was neither cushingoid (symptoms resembling Cushing's syndrome and marked by rapid development of fatty tissue deposits of the face, neck, and trunk, as well as some osteoporosis of the spinal column) nor physically weak anymore. In fact, to all appearances she was totally "normal." She declined medications and refused further testing of her blood or urine, as the *curandera* who treated her had recommended.

She told my medical informant what the old folk healer had done for her. She had been diagnosed with *mal ojo* or evil eye, which had apparently been cast upon her (without her knowledge) by a *brujeria* or witch, who had been hired by a previous, jealous suitor whom the patient spurned in favor of her present boyfriend. This *mal puesto* or witch's hex, it was thought, had brought on her SLE symptoms.

She then explained to her doctor the type of treatment the *curandera* had given her. The old woman made her diagnosis of the hex by rubbing a whole raw egg over the patient's naked body; the egg was then broken open and the yolk carefully examined. A red spot (eye) on the yolk indicated *mal ojo*. The same egg was then placed into a small bowl of water and a cross made of blessed palms laid over it. The patient was then instructed to place it under the head of her bed at night before she went to sleep. This is thought to help draw away the evil force lingering around her as a result of the *brujeria*. The following morning the egg was then buried some distance from the patient's house and away from any plants to avoid the force of any evil from it, perchance wilting them.

The folk healer also gave the young woman a mixture of herbs consisting of equal parts of *aniz verde* (anise seed), *rose de castillo* (rose petals), and *yerba buena* (mint) with instructions to brew them into a warm tea and to drink 3 to 4 cups of it before retiring for the night. The general purpose of the tea was to calm the patient's nerves and help her get over her *susto* or fright sickness incurred as a result of learning about the unsuspecting *brujeria* hex.

During my discussion with the woman's physician about her condition, he seriously doubted that her SLE had "burned out," as he put it. For, as he pointed out to me, at the time of the cessation of medication, histological changes were present on her renal biopsy specimens, her serum complement levels were lower than normal, and the patient's ESRs were "atmospheric" or very high.

But he was at least willing to concede that the placebo benefits obtained from this old *curandera's* treatment defied medical logic, chemical tabulation, or scientific citation. By what mechanism did the machinations of an illiterate *curandera* cure active lupus nephritis, change myxedema into euthyroidism, and permit precipitous withdrawal from corticosteroid treatment without symptoms of adrenal insufficiency?

My medical informant had no answers for these singular phenomena, nor was he prepared to speculate on them either. This then is offered as the best evidence of the "mind over matter" explanation given at the very beginning of this section.

Belief as a Powerful Motivator in Folk Medicine

The subject of belief should be mentioned here. For I am convinced beyond a shadow of doubt that one of the most potent forces at work in any form of practiced folk medicine is a definite belief in the remedies used or methods employed. This *implicit*, almost childlike trust is at the very heart of *curanderismo* and a hundred other alternative medical systems being utilized somewhere worldwide on an hourly or daily basis.

Nothing demonstrates the medical efficacy of this "*complete* freedom from doubt" more than the situation referred to in Numbers 21:5–9. Briefly stated, it is this: As Moses was leading the children of Israel through the wilderness, they rebelled against him and spoke hard words "against God" and himself. Their grumbling had to do with a lack of adequate water and substantial bread, noting how much their souls "loathed this light bread" that was made from the mysterious manna which appeared every morning on the ground and was gathered up by them (see Numbers 11:7–9).

We are next informed that after the people had managed to offend God big-time, that the Lord, in retaliation "sent fiery serpents among [them], and they bit the people, and [many] of Israel died." Realizing their awful error, "the people came to Moses and [apologized saying] we have sinned; [therefore] pray unto the Lord, that he may take away the serpents from us." Moses did as they requested and was told by God to make an image of "a serpent of brass" and to affix it to a very tall pole planted in the ground, so that anyone who had been bitten, "when he [or she] beheld the serpent of brass," was automatically cured and didn't die.

Obviously, both belief *and* faith were simultaneously at work here. Belief in Moses' instruction to look and faith in the image itself were all it took to work a healing miracle. Whether one accepts this Biblical story at its face value or not is beside the point; the fact remains that they were impressed enough with their leader to put absolute trust in what he said.

This same type of confidence was certainly at work with the young lady when she visited that old *curandera* for treatment of her witchcraft-induced systemic lupus erythematosus. I use the term I coined "spiritual homeopathy" for cases like this or the one cited in the Old Testament. For both of them rest on a sound basis in human experience where "like cures like," or wounds heal wounds. The *curandera* practiced a form of "good" witchcraft herself in order to rid her patient of the "bad" witchcraft with which she was then being plagued. The children of Israel had been bitten by desert vipers as punishment for their sins and were of necessity having to look upon an image of the same deadly snakes to find a successful antidote to the venomous toxins circulating in their bodies.

A similar comparison to further illustrate my "spiritual homeopathy" classification is given herewith. In a small town in Maine there lived a young woman who, when a bitter grief came to her, shut herself off from her friends. She refused to be consoled by anyone. One day a saintly old man, also in deep sorrow, came to see her. After they had a good cry together, her broken heart began to mend in an almost miraculous manner, which simply defied logic and explanation, much to the delighted amazement of her family, friends, and several psychotherapists.

In most forms of genuine folk medicine that are practiced in every nation upon the earth, belief and faith are still very much preferred over scientific deduction and medical rationale. This is certainly true when it comes to *curanderismo*. I personally recall an episode which occurred to me back in the early 1970s in the jungles of Guatemala, while on a scientific expedition with some archaeologists. I contracted a severe fever, probably from a mosquito bite, that left me dangerously weak and with temporary mental disorientation. Being far from conventional medical assistance, my colleagues were desperate as to what should be done for my grave situation.

Not far from the archaeological site being worked at stood a small Mayan village in which resided a middle-aged *curandera*. She was recommended by some of the laborers hired from there to do much of the excavation digging. I was carried to her simple hut and laid on the dirt floor, with my friends gathered around me. The woman instructed one of them to squat near me and make sure that I always had plenty of liquid to drink. She then had the others undress me down to my briefs, after which she placed a number of candles on the ground until I was encircled by them. These she lit and then proceeded to gently beat my seminaked body with a branch of moist leaves which she kept dipping in a liquid of some kind. While doing this she prayed to her gods, which were composed of old Mayan deities and Catholic saints. How long this affair went on I don't know, but by the next morning I had regained full consciousness and felt a lot better. My friends admitted upon being questioned later about the matter, that in their fear of losing me, they had set aside enough of their scholastic reasoning to *believe* that this *curandera* might just be able to pull off getting me well again. Nevertheless, upon second reflection later on, they also confessed to thinking that much of what she had uttered over me in her native tongue was gibberish to them, even though that same jabbering nonsense ultimately *cured* me of my terrible condition.

As a trained social scientist specializing in medical anthropology, I've been taught to approach such things with cultural respect but at the same time to view them as coming from primitive minds. On the other hand, as a legitimate folk healer myself and endowed with a "healing intuition" similar to what my grandmother Barbara Leibhardt Heinerman possessed, I've had no choice but to *believe* in the unseen influences which have guided me in many of my own successful treatments.

In fact, *belief* in the supernatural has always been a wonderful and inspiring part of my family's European heritage. My great-grandfather Stefan Heinrich resided in Temesvar, Hungary (now Timisoara,

Romania) in the 1890s. One night he went down to the Danube River to do a little fishing. While there he saw some distance away an old woman come near the river bank and insert a stick into the water with a cloth doll attached to it. Then she picked up a reed and struck the water's surface three times. A horrible-looking spirit arose out of the depths, seized the doll, and tore it to shreds.

After its vicious nature had been somewhat appeased, the woman undertook a conversation with this malovent spirit. Stefan put his fishing rod aside and crept closer to hear what was being said between the two in his native Hungarian. The woman, a well-known witch from those parts, was making an inquiry relative to a local citizen of some wealth and distinction. This fellow had apparently oppressed some poor folks with the weight of the law behind him, and they had come to her to have justice rendered in their behalf. The hideous form growled in a deep voice that he would visit this individual and perform a misery of his own choosing as he has been requested to by her. Satisfied with this, the old witch turned and went away, while the evil spirit vanished into thin air. A few days later Stefan learned that this prominent man had been suddenly seized with a terrible affliction which left him in a great deal of pain; his suffering continued for a short while until he took a turn for the worst and quickly died. To my great-grandfather's superstitious way of thinking, this was a literal fulfillment of what he had been privy to by the riverbank a few weeks before.

My great-grandfather Stefan and his son Jacob Heinerman, Sr. (my grandfather) never got along together; when the latter was old enough to leave home and be on his own, he took his mother's maiden name of Heinerman as his surname and dropped the name of Heinrich which he thoroughly despised. That is how my father's parents brought the name of Heinerman to America, where it remains virtually nonexistent outside of our immediate family circle.

My grandfather's sister Catherine married a fellow by the name of Joseph Wozab. Now the latter had a mother who didn't want her son getting married. Out of jealousy and spite, she consulted with a local gypsy woman who dabbled in the black arts and had a curse placed on him. Soon he began getting thinner and thinner no matter how much he would eat. Alarmed by this condition and fearing for his life, the mother returned to the gypsy and asked that the curse be removed from him.

The gypsy provided her with the instructions to make this happen and Joseph followed them to the letter. He took a live chicken with him to the church cemetery at midnight, where he then released it into the air. He then turned around and walked away without looking back. He suddenly heard a loud screech from the bird, followed by a distinctive pop or exploding sound. The next morning he returned to the graveyard and discovered bits of chicken guts and feathers scattered over a circumference of several feet, while dried chicken blood stained a number of tombstones within the same area. But after this strange incident, he soon regained his former weight and never had another problem like this again.

As mentioned before, one of the central themes in folk medicine everywhere is the belief in witchcraft and sorcery, which come in two basic flavors, good (white magic) and bad (black magic). All of them use common elements in different combinations—candles, incense, prayers, dolls to which an article of the beneficiary or victim is attached, and other things as well. The Christian cross as heavily exemplified in Catholicism is frequently used also.

But all of these magical objects and the powers by which they work require the belief and faith of those performing them, as well as that of those who've made the requests for such. *Curanderismo* is no different in this respect and commands an abiding trust in the supernatural in order to be fully functional.

A Curandero in Action: One Day in the Life of a Mexican-American Folk Healer

There is a great scene near the end of the classic Western *The Horse Soldiers* (1959) starring John Wayne and William Holden that pretty well typifies the attitudes of many average Mexican-Americans toward the medical profession in general. Wayne is telling a woman his opinion about surgeons: "I seen a young girl the same age as that boy that just died. She was operated on by doctors, too. It was a tumor they said and had to come out. So I let two of them work on her, while I held her down. They put a piece of leather into her mouth so she could bite her screams away. Well, they cut her open all right and found nothing, I tell you, nothing at all wrong with her. Oh, they said they was sorry all right after she died. But what about me? What about me? I once had faith in them but not no more!"

In the time I spent along both sides of the river in the Lower Rio Grande Valley of southern Texas and northern Mexico, I had ample opportunities presented me to interview several hundred different patients belonging to a few prominent practitioners of *curanderismo* there. Almost to a person they told me of their general distrust in regular *medicos* or doctors, and instead preferred the services of someone like Hector Salinas, a respected faith healer with whom I was privileged to sit and observe while quietly taking notes as he conducted his practice from within his own home.

On one typical morning, there were six people (four women and two men) waiting to see him. We sat with a timid young lady named Margarita Estrada in a side room. She spoke softly, almost reverently. After Hector had asked why she hadn't consulted a medical doctor, she responded that she didn't hold any confidence in them whatsoever, that all they wanted was her money, and did very little to actually help a person. He then asked her to tell him what her anxieties were all about.

After listening for about ten minutes, this *curandero* scribbled a prescription on a common physician's pad. He instructed her to place two lighted white candles on a table and place a glass of water between them. Under the water glass she was told to put a photograph of herself. Salinas also prescribed *manzanilla* or chamomile tea, of which she had to drink 3 cups daily for 4 days straight.

We watched as Ms. Estrada folded the prescription and carefully tucked it in her purse. She seemed pleased by what he had just given her and laid two crinkled dollar bills on the table in front of her as a "donation" to the *curandero*. He told me afterward that he never charges for his counsel, but that within their culture it is customary to leave a gift offering of some kind for the time that was spent with an individual.

"I gave her *manzanilla* to calm her nerves and give her strength of mind," Salinas said later. "She thinks she will lose her job, so we give her some preventative help. . . . Many, many, many people that come to see me say they can't cope with their jobs. That is the most frequent complaint I get."

The candles and water mostly are symbolic gestures, he noted. When I asked him about how many of his compatriots visit *curanderos* like him regularly, he guessed about seven out of every ten—an estimate pretty close to those I got from other practitioners of *curanderismo* in the Valley.

Before receiving what he called "the gift of healing" in 1978, Salinas was an Hidalgo County deputy sheriff. I remember my informant as a big man with black wavy hair, a protruding girth, and a very piercing stare. He claimed he was a Christian and a *"curandero muy bueno"*—very good folk healer. Some healers, he noted, work with the black arts and can do as much harm as good.

The next patient in was a wizened, middle-aged man with an obvious alcohol problem (he fairly reeked of tequila). Hector recommended an herb called *haba de San Ignacio (Hura crepitans)*. He got up and walked over to a cupboard against one wall, opened the doors, and took from it a small coffee can, out of which he measured so much powdered haba beans. This he scooped into a brown bag and gave it to the alcoholic with instructions to add one teaspoonful to his meals. (Hector let me in on a little secret after his patient had exited the room about his choice of remedy for the man. "These beans will induce vomiting if he takes a drink of tequila with his meal," he said with a sly smile. "He doesn't know that but will soon find out if he uses alcohol when he eats. The main purpose of this little remedy is to get him to quit on his own without him knowing that the haba beans were responsible for doing this.")

Hector then removed from the cupboard a broken shard of green glass that had once been part of an old Coca Cola bottle. He held it in the palm of his cupped right hand and stared into it with his hard and intense gaze. His face took on a more serious look as he informed the slightly inebriated patient: "I see by my crystal that if you do not mend your ways soon, *mi amigo,* you will die like a dog in the streets somewhere and be given a pauper's burial without even a priest to administer last rites over you!" This piece of unhappy news hit the old gent pretty hard and a tear or two rolled down his unshaven cheeks as he contemplated a death without a priest's final blessings and worried about his hapless soul drifting off into Purgatory as a result of this.

He slowly stood up, wiped away the moisture from his face with the back of one hand, took the sack with powdered beans, dropped some coin change on the table, shook Hector's hand, and then shuffled out of the room. Hector explained his rationale for using the crystal here but not with the first patient: "This man needed a strong vision to warn him of impending circumstances if he doesn't change. I spoke what I saw and think it may help him. Who knows, though, how he'll turn out? You try your best but it's still up to them to want to change."

The next person into the little room was a woman named Mariana, somewhere in her forties, who stood on her feet for most of the day in *maquiladoras* across the border in Matamores, where she assembled components for Motorola cell phones. After some initial inquiry on Hector's part, she finally told him her problem: Her feet had been bothering her for some months now and she wanted some relief.

He went to his cupboard and brought out a can of WD-40 and ordered her to remove her shoes and stockings. He dragged his chair around in front of her, sat down, and lifted one leg up, placing it on his lap. He sprayed a little of the WD-40 in between her toes and on the bottom of her sole, as well as a little into the palms of his hands. He then began massaging the bottom of her foot in circular, clockwise motions. After five minutes on that foot, he switched to the other one for the same length of time. He then got a wet hand towel and rubbed off any excess WD-40 so as not to cause a rash.

The woman got up, put her stockings and shoes back on, walked around the room a bit, and said her feet no longer ached. He wrote out a simple prescription for two cans of WD-40 with instructions to her husband on how to use it each night on his wife's feet, and handed it to her. She placed a crisp ten-dollar bill on the table, smiled, and waved a fond farewell as she walked out. "I usually don't get donations that large," he replied, "and will sometimes protest if I know the person can't afford it. But in her case, both she and her husband work and make pretty good money between them, and this is what she feels is adequate for the service I performed."

In all of my years of folk medicine investigations, I had never seen nor heard of WD-40 being used for something like this. My informant shrugged off my amazement by deliberately *understating* the remedy's success: "It's really nothing to get excited about. The *curanderos* down here like myself use it fairly often to beat arthritis, relieve stiff necks and shoulders, get rid of backaches, and bring comfort to sore muscles."

He suggests the 9-ounces size because of its carrying convenience, and always advises his patients to try a little on a small area of skin before spraying it over a large portion. Should a rash develop, as sometimes happens with those having sensitive skin, then they should not be using it too frequently, only when needed the most for quick relief. "It won't hurt the skin that much," he said, "but it's good to be cautious anyway."

After this came an older woman (probably in her sixties we estimated) accompanied by a young teenage girl with a bright smile. As they seated themselves opposite Hector, the girl introduced herself as Lola and the woman beside her. "This is my grandmother, who doesn't speak much English and asked that I come with her to help translate."

Hector turned around and flashed me a quick grin, as if to suggest he was willing to go along with the little "joke." "I *do* speak fluent Spanish," he informed the girl with a smile. She quickly sized up the situation and replied, "Oh no, it's not that, *señor*. You misunderstood me. I'm here to translate for my grandmother because she is full-blooded *Indian* and only speaks Tarahumara." Hector glanced my way again and this time it was my turn to grin, as the "joke" was now on him.

After much back-and-forth discussion, it turned out that the old lady's problem was severe headaches. She had tried different things, including aspirin, but nothing seemed to work. Hector told her through the granddaughter that the *remedio* was a very simple one. With that, he got up and walked through a back door into his kitchen to fetch a potato. He returned with a medium-sized Idaho baker and proceeded to cut it into thick slices on the table in front of them.

"Papas are very good for making things like this disappear," he told the girl, who then translated that and everything else he said. Acting on his instructions, the old woman arose from her chair and went over and lay down on an old couch against a far wall. Hector pulled a red bandanna out of his back pocket and tied it around her forehead. He slipped slices of raw potato in between where the throbbing was the most pronounced—typically at the forehead and temples. Next, he tightened the bandanna a little more to achieve a slight pressure, then had her close her eyes and lie there awhile. The three of us—Hector, myself, and the young girl—then left the room for about an hour.

Outside he chatted amiably with the remaining patients waiting to see him, two women and a man. The latter suffered from asthma and the *remedio* prescribed for his condition struck me as being really odd, if not "off-the-wall" a little. Hector advised him to get a Mexican Chihuahua and keep it near him at all times, especially when he slept. "This will take away your problem," he reassured the fellow. Sometime after this I had occasion to visit a veterinarian friend of mine and told him about this most unusual remedy. He laughed and said, "That's more folklore than folk medicine." He then explained what was probably the rationale behind Hector's suggestion. Small dogs (Yorkshire terriers and toy poodles, as well as Chihuahuas) have tiny tracheas that tend to collapse as the dogs age. When this happens, the tracheal rings then vibrate with every breath, and the dogs usually have trouble breathing. In the medical lore of Mexican American *curanderismo,* this respiratory problem becomes the "asthma" that the dog presumably can "take away" from its master.

But if this one belongs in the realm of medical fiction, then the rest of Hector's suggestions certainly were based in solid facts. One of the two remaining women suffered from a bad case of the hiccups.

He excused himself for a moment and went around to the back side of his house (so as not to disturb the older patient resting on the couch inside) to get some dry granulated sugar and a spoon from his kitchen. He returned with the items and had this person slowly swallow a teaspoonful of the sugar. The hiccuping became less frequent. He had her take another spoonful the same way, and within a minute or two after doing this, her hiccuping had ceased altogether. She gave a donation of one dollar, hugged him, and went away completely satisfied with the results. A while later I asked a doctor friend about this, whose specialty is otolargyngology (ear-nose-throat). His explanation was something to this effect: The granules of sugar can irritate the throat (pharynx), thus interfering with the impulses of the vagus nerve, which trigger spasms of the diaphragm that result in incessant hiccuping. He had never heard of this particular remedy before, but assumed that it would work better than other strategies for the reason just given.

The last woman stated that she was there on behalf of her father, who was at home suffering from a very nasty cold. They were too poor to afford conventional prescription antibiotics and she was sent to find out what inexpensive *remedios* could be used in their place. Hector suggested that she make a simple soup broth and include "pinches" of grated horseradish root, cayenne pepper, and powdered cloves, which when he ate some of this, would unclog him in no time and "make a new man out of him." (Some of the volatile chemical constituents in such spices appear to stimulate production of watery secretions in the lungs, which makes it easier to cough up phlegm. But be advised to use such strong spices *in moderation!*)

By now over an hour had passed and everyone else had gone except for the Indian grandmother resting peacefully inside.

We went back into the room and Hector gently roused her from her light slumber. He then removed the bandanna and potato slices from her head. She sat up and declared in her native tongue that her headache was *totally gone!* A customary donation was offered, verbal gratitude expressed, and both women left obviously pleased with the results. I walked over to the table and felt some of the potato slices; they seemed hot and dry to my touch. Hector explained that *papas* are very good for absorbing the heat generated at these particular pressure points; though he didn't understand anything about Chinese medicine, I suspected that principles of acupressure were at work here.

"A really good *curandero* never solicits business," Hector reminded me. "My business flourishes only on my reputation as a folk healer. If I am successful most of the time, then people will spread it far and wide. I average five to seven patients a day, five days a week. Many of them are first-timers who have heard about me from word-of-mouth. Sometimes if I get a difficult case I know I can't cure, such as a paralytic, I will tell them so in the very beginning so there is no misunderstanding between us. *El Señor Dios* [God] has given me a great gift and I try to act wisely and honestly whenever I use it. *That* is the mark of a good *curandero.*"

Remedios Caseros: Home Remedies from Hispanic Barrios Throughout America

While the bulk of my ethnographic research centered on both sides of the border in the Lower Rio Grande Valley of southern Texas in 1985, I also had other occasions later on to work with folk healers in various parts of Florida and in the Spanish Harlem section of Manhattan in New York City. They provided additional data which proved worthwhile in my studies.

All of the information that was gathered from these several different sources was eventually compiled and added to this particular section. I believe that the whole of it greatly enriches the chapter and adds to our overall understanding and appreciation for the many wonderful contributions which Hispanic Americans from throughout the Western Hemisphere have made to the folk medicine which our nation has been marvelously endowed with.

I've arranged these *remedios caseros* in the order of their popularity, given both their Spanish and English names, and briefly mentioned some of the ethnopharmacological treatments for which they've been utilized.

MANZANILLA/Chamomile (*Matricaria chamomilla*).   In the Lower Rio Grande Valley the fresh or dried leafy stems and flowers are made into a warm tea and taken to allay stomach distress and nausea. Throughout Puerto Rico, the dried plant, broken into small pieces, is sold in plastic bags. This is one of the most used of all *remedios caseros* in that American commonwealth. In El Salvador the tea has been used to treat *susto* (soul fright), one of the most prevailing folk illnesses of magical origin indigenous to all of Latin America.

SAVILA/Aloe Vera (*Aloe barbadensis*).   This has the widest variety of uses of all of the core *remedios* of the different *curanderos y curanderas* whom I interviewed. The raw, clear sap obtained from breaking part of a leaf off and squeezing it out between the fingers has been used topically to treat burns, sunburns, cuts, skin sores, acne, infected wounds, skin ulcers, shingles, eczema, dermatitis, athlete's foot, herpes sores. It is also added to hot water or hot milk sweetened with sugar, and gargled to relieve sore throats and coughs.

RUDA/Rue (*Ruta graveolens*).   Cuban-American practitioners of *curanderismo* largely depend on a decoction made of the leaves to induce or increase menstrual flow; it is taken on an empty stomach in the A.M. and a second time in the P.M. It is also given to pregnant women when they are due to minimize labor pains and maximize delivery. Some Salvadoran folk healers in the Miami and New York City areas use the expressed juice of heated fresh leaves when lukewarm as ear drops to overcome earache. A decoction of 10 grams (⅓ ounce) in 250 cc (approx. ⅔ pint) water will kill lice effectively.

YERBA ANIZ/Anise (*Pimpinella anisum*).   Cuban-American folk healers commonly use an alcoholic infusion of the aromatic fruit to relieve intestinal gas and extreme heartburn. Twenty grams (⅔ ounce) of anise fruit is steeped in one pint of alcohol (rum) for this purpose. A little swig is taken after a heavy meal. In Lima, Peru, a decoction of 4 grams fruit (¼ ounce) in 160 cc (less than ½ pint) is taken 4 times daily as a tonic and to promote breast milk in nursing mothers.

YERBA BUENA/Mint (*Mentha spicata*). Colombian folk healers in Dade County, Florida, make a warm tea of the leaves to stop vomiting, dispel heart palpitations, and "cure" stomach cancer. Salvadorans in New York's Spanish Harlem district will often use poultices made of the fresh, cooked leaves to relieve rheumatic pains and on the forehead and about the temples to get rid of migraines. Peruvian immigrants to America still use an old Inca remedy for getting rid of athlete's feet and foot odor by soaking their feet in a footbath made from the leaves. Virtually all Latin American immigrants whom I interviewed use mint leaf tea as a skin wash for sores, to stop diarrhea in kids, and to reduce fevers.

ESTAFIATE/Wormwood (*Artemisia mexicana*). A remedy probably carried over from Spain a long time ago is prevalent throughout New York's Spanish Harlem. A strong decoction is made and rubbed on rheumatic joints to relieve pain and stiffness. The root is used as a tea to expel intestinal parasites and given in known cases of epilepsy to reduce the number of seizures.

FRUTA DE LIMA Y HOJAS DE LIMA/Lime fruit and lime tree leaves (*Citrus aurantium*). This is a very popular remedy among all Latin American folk healers (including those who've immigrated to the United States). The juice in hot water stops diarrhea. It is flushed into the nostrils to stop nosebleeds. Diluted in hot water, it is gargled for throat infections. The juice of 2 freshly squeezed limes in an 8-ounce glass of cool water is taken to reduce fevers, treat liver complaints, and eliminate edema. A great remedy for diabetes that *really works* calls for the juice of fresh limes to be taken by straw each day to avoid harming tooth enamel: the juice of 1 lime on the first day, of 2 on the second day, and soon until the juice of 18 to 20 limes total has been ingested. Then cut back the dose to 1 lime per day again and commence the routine anew. The peel of 3 limes is boiled for 10 minutes in 1 quart water and then refrigerated. One cup is taken daily. Either of these remedies will reduce blood sugar levels very nicely. I've interviewed Hispanic diabetics who claim these have worked for them.

ALBACAR/Sweet basil (*Ocimum basilicum*).   Some Salvadorans will stuff fresh leaves into the ears as a sure remedy for deafness. Cuban-Americans make a dinner decoction of the fresh or dried leaves to help digest their food. Colombian *curanderas* in New York City apply the crushed leaves as a frontal poultice to allay headaches. And Puerto Ricans in Manhattan have been known to drink copious amounts of the leaf tea prior to random urinalysis checks for illegal drugs in the blood. (Basil quickly removes any trace of drug residue in the blood or urine.)

OREGANO/Oregano/marjoram   (*Monarda   menthaefolia*). Some Peruvian folk healers in South Florida make an infusion of the fresh herb to help settle an upset stomach; relieve a headache; get rid of colic; calm jittery nerves due to caffeine, nicotine, alcohol, or illicit drugs; relieve coughing; reduce abdominal cramps in women and regulate their menstrual cycle when taken 4 days before their normal periods begin; prevent motion and morning sicknesses; and facilitate breathing in cases of asthma and bronchitis.

AJO/Garlic (*Allium sativum*).   Chewing a garlic clove every day is a standard recommendation with nearly all folk healers throughout Latin America and in the Hispanic barrios of the United States. By doing so, they claim, a person will never get sick, will never look old, and live to be a hundred or more. It is standard folk therapy for diabetes (but not recommended by me for those with existing hypoglycemia). To expel intestinal worms, crush 1 or 2 cloves and boil in milk or lemon juice, then drink lukewarm. Many Hispanics will wear or carry with them a bulb of garlic when attending a funeral or visiting a cemetery to ward off *espiritos malos* (bad spirits). Cuban-American folk healers apply the crushed garlic cloves to the sites of scorpion stings, centipede bites, and spider bites to reduce swelling and draw out the poison. I once saw a victim of a deadly brown recluse spider bite treating exclusively for 10 days with nothing but garlic internally and externally and *fully recovered!* Now *that* is a testament to the healing powers of garlic!

PELOS DE ELOTE/Corn silks (*Zea mays*). Immigrants from Costa Rica residing in Los Angeles County make a strong decoction of corn silk to treat infectious hepatitis that comes from consuming food prepared by food handlers already infected with the disease. It is not uncommon to find little heaps of the dried, red-brown cornsilk in stores in South Miami that sell medicinal herbs to numerous Hispanic customers; they buy this a lot to make a tea for "kidney trouble." The tea is sweetened and drunk in place of water to dissolve bladder and kidney stones. Two Colombian and one Venezuelan folk healer who ply their trades in New Jersey use *both* the silk and the husks of corn in a strong decoction to successfully halt menstrual bleeding. A common Mexican aphrodisiac for waning sexual prowess calls for roasting a half-ripe ear of corn *before* it is dehusked, the husk removed afterward, and the ear placed in a wide-mouthed jar with some rusty nails. The bottle is filled with brandy and then let set. Six ounces of this is drunk 3 times daily before bedroom activity begins.

CANELA/Cinnamon (*Cinnamomum zeylanicum*). Puerto Rican folk healers make a strong tea out of cinnamon sticks to kill germs and bacteria in the mouth that cause gum disease, cavities, and bath breath, in the lungs and throat that bring on colds and flus, in the stomach that may induce nausea and vomiting, and in the colon where they can cause diarrhea.

ROMERO/Rosemary (*Rosmarinus officinalis*). A strong decoction made of the leafy stems and flowers is sometimes recommended by a few practitioners of *curanderismo* to achieve abortion and induce temporary sterility in men. An alcoholic infusion of 20 grams (slightly less than an ounce) with 10 grams (about ½ ounce) of dried lavender is applied on contusions and sprains and rubbed on the scalp to stop falling hair. Cuban-Americans seem to prefer the fresh plant over the dried, and use it for treating insomnia, nervousness, heart pain, asthma and bronchitis, and hysteria when taken as a *wine* infusion (wine used in place of water to make a tea with).

BORRAJA/Borage (*Borago officinalis*). Salvadoran immigrants like to use the mucilaginous juice of the fresh plant to induce or increase perspiration in fevers as well as to reduce them. Colombian nationals who practice folk medicine in Florida prescribe a tea made of 10 grams (⅓ ounce) leaves boiled/steeped in 100 grams (3½ ounce) water for edema, and as an eyewash to dispel red eye and inflammation when the solution is diluted.

CENIZO/Purple sage (*Leucophyllum texanun*).   Puerto Rican, Guatemalan, and Mexican immigrants use the plant decoction for indigestion and rheumatism. The crushed leaves are poulticed on wounds to hasten healing by Cuban American *curanderos*. Panamanian and Peruvian nationals drink the tea for hypertension and to get rid of colds. Colombian mothers make a decoction to wash their children's skin to relieve the itching and inflammation accompanying measles and chickenpox.

NOPAL/Prickly pear cactus (*Opuntia* spp.).   Texas *curanderos* split the joints open and use the mucilaginous flesh as an effective poultice on toothache, earache, erysipelas, rheumatism, inflamed eyes, sunburns, burns, and on the abdomen and over the liver to reduce internal inflammation and halt diarrhea. The split, cooked joint is sometimes poulticed on abscesses to help draw out purulent matter. An infusion of the mucilaginous flesh is used as an effective scalp shampoo to stimulate new hair growth.

ROSA DE CASTILLO/Rose (*Rosa centifolia*).   There are over 100 species of roses, and to them and their varieties have been given thousands of names. In the face of such abundance, it may be best to say with Shakespeare's Juliet" "What's in a name? That which we call a rose / By any other name would smell as sweet." Peruvian nationals make a decoction of the petals by simmering them for 10 minutes to treat canker sores inside the mouth and on the tongue (they hold the cool tea inside and swish it around for up to 2 minutes). A wine decoction invigorates a tired body and exhausted mind.

SALVIA/Sage (*Salvia leucantha*).   Cuban-Americans bind the fresh leaves on the head to relieve headache and reduce fever. I watched one Venezuelan folk healer in New York's famed Spanish

Harlem district crush some fresh leaves in a mortar with a stone pestle and then rub it onto the skin between the ear and chin of an older woman to relieve her facial neuralgia. A Guatemalan folk healer in the Lower Rio Grande Valley of south Texas heated some fresh leaves in hot water and then applied them as an effective styptic to the nicks and abrasions on her teenage grandson's face incurred while he hastily and carelessly shaved himself with a new razor blade. Swelling of any body part is treated with a strong tea made of the leafy branch tip by Peruvian nationals.

HOJAS DE MESQUITE/Mesquite leaves (*Prosopis glandulosa*). A leaf decoction is used as a mouth rinse and when a tooth abscess is bursting by Mexican-Americans. They also finely mash the leaves, mix in brown sugar, and make an eye salve to dispel inflammation.

MARIJUANA/Marijuana (*Cannabis sativa*). It is unfortunate that this plant is still banned by the federal government on account of its extensive use as an illicit drug. I have long been a proponent of its *medicinal* uses for *legitimate* health reasons. This plant, in spite of its current illegal status because of government prejudice and stupidity, is still widely utilized by many Hispanic *curanderas* in the United States. In cases of extreme mental anguish or profound melancholy that may border on near suicidal, the leaf is smoked in cigarette form in what is known on the streets as a "joint." This helps to relax the highly agitated mind of the patient so that he or she can be properly reasoned with through counseling. Usually no more than half a joint needs to be smoked to achieve this purpose. In the severe migraines accompanying brain tumors, joint smoking affords tremendous relief and makes the cancer patient's life a great deal easier. It is good for combating nervous trembling and reducing the number of seizures in epilepsy.

NOGAL/Pecan (*Carya illonoensis*). A few Mexican American and Puerto Rican *curanderos* advise their obese patients to snack on pecans as a great way to lose some weight and feel more energetic. Borrowing on their idea, I've made it one of the chief snack foods in my own weight-loss diet, which has helped individuals lose an average of 5 to 7 pounds per week while on the diet. Slivered pecans mixed with some water in a food blender make a delicious nut milk for those who don't wish to drink dairy products.

COMINO/Cumin (*Arracacia atropurpurea*). Nursing mothers among the Colombian nationals living in New York and Florida drink a leaf decoction to promote the flow of breast milk. The seeds are eaten and the leaves rubbed on the face and body by some Puerto Rican immigrants in hopes of lightening the hue of their skin. Salvadorans make a tea from the seeds to relieve intestinal gas and heartburn. Cuban-Americans make a tea of the aromatic and pungent seeds to treat testicular inflammation.

SACATE DE LIMON/Lemon grass (*Cymbopogon citratus*). Costa Rican folk healers in the United States use an infusion of the rhizome as a mouthwash to cure pyorrhea of the gums. Cuban-Americans drink an infusion of the roots and leaves to overcome colds and cases of influenza.

EL AZAJAR/Orange blossoms/orange peel/orange juice (*Citrus sinensis*). Peruvian nationals still use the tree blossoms steeped in warm water as a pleasant sedative for nervousness and insomnia. Colombian nationals use the leaf infusion or decoction as an antispasmodic for hysteria, heart palpitations, convulsions, and seizures. In Spanish Harlem, a decoction of orange peel is a remedy for intestinal worms and gas. Freshly squeezed juice from half an orange is rubbed on the tongue to combat thrush.

CEBOLLA/Onion (*Allium cepa*). Spanish folk medicine includes many remedies that utilize this important culinary spice. The freshly squeezed juice is applied on severe burns to help heal them. To expel intestinal worms, a fasting person drinks water in which a chopped-up onion has soaked overnight or white wine in which a crushed onion soaked for 6 days. A dose of 4 spoonfuls of onion juice daily has been claimed by numerous *curanderos y curanderas* to cure epilepsy. Onion juice and vinegar are mixed and rubbed on the faces of teenagers to eliminate many of their pimples. An onion infusion is taken to relieve stubborn coughs, edema, and stones in the kidneys or gallbladder. Sliced onion is bound over the ear with flannel to relieve an earache and ringing in the ear. Mashed onion bulb is applied directly on the sites of spider bites and scorpion stings, as well as wasp, hornet, and bee stings. Onion juice, sweetened with sugar, is given to young children to expel intestinal worms. A strong onion decoction is used as an effective remedy for chest colds and tuberculosis.

OLIVO/Olive (*Simarouba glauca*).   Cuban-Americans use the bitter leaves and bark in decoctions for treating venereal diseases, herpes simplex, and AIDS.

TORONJIL/Lemon balm (*Melissa officinalis*).   Salvadoran folk healers apply the leaf decoction to wounds, bruises, and skin ulcers. An infusion of the leaves, taken one cup with each meal, promotes digestion and dispels gas. The infusion is drunk several times a day as an antispasmodic and remedy for heart palpitations and coronary pain due to angina. Puerto Ricans in America like the warm leaf infusion as a wonderful nerve tonic and terrific sedative for agitation, hysteria, and migraine headaches. A warm decoction given rectally as an enema will halt bloody diarrhea. Peruvian nationals in Los Angeles County place fresh leaves on the eyelids and use the plant decoction as an eyewash to relieve eye inflammation.

LIMON/Lemon (*Citrus aurantifolia*).   Cuban-Americans in South Florida take lemon juice straight or diluted with water for coughs and colds. For persistent coughing, a teaspoon of lemon juice and honey (equal parts) is mixed, held in the mouth, and then slowly swallowed.

MALVA/Mallow (*Malva parviflora*).   Salvadorans in Spanish Harlem drink a decoction made from the root to treat fevers and chickenpox in young children. Other Hispanic *curanderos y curanderas* regard the plant as a cure-all. They drink the decoction to reduce fever, promote menstrual flow, and clean up pneumonia. The mashed leaves, with salt and vinegar or with sugar, are applied on the temples to allay a headache. Hispanic mothers who've just given birth will drink the decoction (sometimes sweetened with brown sugar), or eat the fresh or dry leaves after cooking them with raisins in water for an hour, for the first 3 days following childbirth. The plant decoction is also used for bathing skin eruptions. Chilean-American women use this same remedy as an effective vaginal douche.

GRANADA/Pomegranate (*Punica granatum*). Colombian and Puerto Rican nationals make a decoction of the fruit and rind to stop diarrhea, dysentery, and pneumonia, and to expel tapeworms. This same decoction is good for hemorrhoids and a sore throat.

TELA DE ARANA/Spider web. Mexican-American *curanderos y curanderas* use handfuls of cobwebs to stop minor bleeding. A handful of cobwebs is also mixed with 2 tablespoons of tincture of witch hazel and applied over sunburns to reduce inflammation and itching. Spun spider webs may also be gathered and mixed with a tiny amount of petroleum jelly and applied to bedsores with good results.

TOMATES/Tomatoes (*Physalis ixocarpa*). The tomato is one of the world's leading fruit-vegetables, but in midnineteenth-century America was still considered a poisonous plant by many people. Salvadoran nationals apply the ripe fruit pulp to inflamed hemorrhoids. Cuban-Americans place the tomato slices on burns to eliminate pain and prevent blistering. Tomato juice with a pinch of cayenne pepper added to it will revive the liver and give a boost of much-needed physical energy. The cut, green fruit is applied on ringworm and eaten to cure a sore throat and expel intestinal worms.

MARRUBIO/Horehound (*Marrubium vulgare*). Hispanic folk healers occasionally employ this herb as an expectorant to remove mucus accumulation in the back of the throat and in the lungs. It relieves hoarseness. For fevers, it is unsurpassed. An infusion of the entire herb is made and then taken while still warm.

MIEL Y LIMON/Honey and lemon.   This is probably one of the oldest folk remedy standbys in numerous cultures, be they of Hispanic, Asiatic, European, Native American, African, Oceanic, on Indian origin. The typical ratio is usually a 1:4 with 1 teaspoon *warm* on melted honey mixed in with 4 tablespoons freshly squeezed lemon juice. It makes a fantastic gargle for sore throats and relieves hoarseness. It is good in cases of asthma and bronchitis to facilitate better breathing. It clears up canker sores and gum disease inside the mouth when held there for a minute or so and gently swished around with the tongue.

NUEZ MOSCADA/Nutmeg (*Myristica fragrans*).   The spice improves appetite and digestion when mixed with certain foods. It is a popular remedy with Hispanics.

YERBA AMARILLA/Sunflower (*Helianthus* spp.).   Colombian folk healers recommend that a decoction be made of the bright yellow flowers for weakness of the heart. Peruvian *curanderos y curanderas* suggest an infusion of the leaves for any type of stomach distress; the fresh leaves are applied directly to the skin to soothe it in cases of inflammation like sunburn. Some Costa Rican immigrants will use the flower decoction to relieve fever and cold. And Mexican-Americans will sometimes extract the juice from the flowers and seeds by means of a press, which is reputed to be a "remedio mucho grande" for intermittent fever, edema, cancer, palsy, and stones in the gallbladder and kidneys.

AGUACATE/Avocado (*Persea americana*).   Some Puerto Rican immigrants have boiled 6 leaves or a few pieces of bark (or both together) from the tree in 1 quart of water; the decoction is sweetened, strained, and taken at the rate of 4 tablespoonfuls every 2 hours as a useful remedy for coughs, chronic inflammation of a mucous membrane, or delayed menstruation. Mexican-American practitioners of *curanderismo* make an infusion from 6 tree leaves and a piece of the seed in 1 pint of water, which is then strained and sweetened; 2 tablespoonfuls are then given every 2 hours to patients suffering from diarrhea. Salvadorans and Cuban-Americans make an infusion of avocado tree leaves to remove excess fluid accumulations in body tissues and mucus buildup in the lungs. Colombian nationals in South Florida make a strong decoction of the leaves of the green-skinned avocados to lower blood pressure. Venezuelans transplanted to Los Angeles County heat the tree leaves and apply them to the forehead to relieve a headache; they bind fresh leaves on the feet to reduce fever. One tablespoon of the fresh, grated avocado rind or peel is steeped in 8 ounces of hot seltzer water for 10 minutes, sweetened with a pinch of sugar, stirred, and taken on an empty stomach for 2 days to expel intestinal parasites. The avocado pit can be chopped up, toasted, and pulverized and used as a poultice to get rid of hemorrhoids and herpes sores.

ALCANFOR/Camphor (*Cinnamomum camphora*). Camphor is sometimes utilized by Hispanic folk healers for different problems, but not that often. It has been used externally as a wash, liniment, or ointment for skin ulcers, gangrene, scabies, sprains, bruises, rheumatic pains, and convulsions. I was witness to one Colombian *curandero* working out of his home in Miami, Florida, who treated migraines and assorted neuralgic pains by applying a small amount of camphor to a handkerchief or piece of clean flannel and rubbing it on the forehead and temples (headache) or between the ears and jaw (neuralgia). The same person applied some of it directly to the foot of one patient to treat the pain of an ingrown toenail (relief was almost instantaneous). Camphor is also beneficial to use on herpes sores and superficially for erysipelas.

ALTAMISA/Mugwort (*Artemisia vulgaris*).   Puerto Rican Americans use a bitter decoction of the flowering branches to treat fevers, worms, female problems, and nervous disorders (including epilepsy).

ALFALFA/Alfalfa.   Generally recommended in tea form by many Hispanic folk doctors for improving the appetite, relieving urinary and bowel problems, eliminating retained water, and even helping to cure peptic ulcers.

SODA DE MARTILLO/Baking soda (*Sodium bicarbonate*).
Somewhat popular with Peruvian immigrants, who sprinkle it on sunburned skin to relieve the pain, reduce the inflammation, and prevent excessive peeling. It is also mixed with water or milk and drunk for intestinal gas, kidney stones, suppressed urine, and general poisoning. It is also sprinkled on the skin to relieve severe itching.

CILANTRO/Coriander (*Coriandrum sativum*).   Salvadorans chew the round and ribbed fruits and swallow them to improve digestion and to avoid formation of intestinal gas or heartburn following heavy meals. Puerto Ricans boil 1 tablespoonful of fruit in ½ quart wine, steep, strain, and drink for worms and delayed menstruation. Cuban-Americans take the fruit decoction for neuralgia and diabetes .

HOJAS DE GUAYAVA/Guava leaves (*Psidium guajava*).
Venezuelan immigrants take the leaf decoction to relieve gastroenteritis and diarrhea; they also use it for soaking swollen legs. Guatemalan, Colombian, and Peruvian nationals make a decoction of the leaves—1 ounce of leaves in ½ pint of boiling water—and sweeten it with a little sugar before taking at the rate of ½ cup every 2 hours to overcome diarrhea and intestinal colic. Without sweetening, it is used to bathe mange in animals and for fistulas and skin ulcers. The dried, powdered leaves are applied to skin ulcers and ringworm with good success. A leaf decoction is employed for bathing bed sores and herpes sores. Mexican Americans utilize both the leaf and the bark decoction for relieving stomach pains. Some Panamanian immigrants use a leaf decoction as a wash to treat skin diseases ranging from shingles, psoriasis, and eczema in adults to measles, mumps, and chickenpox in kids. The ripe fruit is eaten to overcome respiratory problems. And some of the fruit juice (1 cup) is drunk with each meal to relieve hiatal hernia.

HUEVOS/Eggs.   Raw egg is a common remedy employed by practitioners of *curanderismo* to treat *mal de ojo*, a widely occurring folk illness throughout all of Latin America and found in most Hispanic *barrios* (neighborhoods) in America. The raw egg is used mostly for ritual reasons in the banishment of this "evil eye" phenomena. Note, however, that raw eggs may be contaminated with *Salmonella*, a bacteria that causes food poisoning.

LECHUGA/Lettuce (*Lactuca sativa*). Colombian nationals employ a leaf decoction of ordinary iceberg lettuce for any kidney, bladder, or urinary difficulties that they may be experiencing. Venezuelan and Guatemalan immigrants use the same decoction to relieve coughs and bronchial asthma. Mexican-Americans find that a decoction made from a strong type of lettuce, such as Romaine or endive, will act as a mild sedative to overcome insomnia. Panamanians know that eating a lettuce salad about 30 minutes before retiring will virtually guarantee a good night's sleep. And Cuban-Americans in Miami take an infusion of the leaves to relieve the severe pain accompanying angina and to correct heart palpitations.

MEJORANA/Marjoram (*Majorana hortensis*). Mexican-American folk healers find marjoram infusions to be very helpful for reducing fevers, clearing up stomachaches, and stopping diarrhea. Venezuelan immigrants make a *warm* decoction for treating mucus accumulation in the lungs, calming hysteria, stopping epileptic seizures, and overcoming alcoholic drunkenness. The warm tea is drunk on an empty stomach in the morning and again at night to banish pain in the side. Hot baths of the fresh leaf decoction are claimed to relieve muscular pain common to sports injuries and heavy physical labor, as well as rheumatism. Cuban-Americans use the decoction to dispel flatulence and to ease the pain of delivery for women in labor (in the latter situation it is almost always given quite *warm*). Sometimes orange peel and anise will be added to the marjoram leaf decoction to enhance the medicinal benefits. Brazilian-Americans like to place the mashed leaves over the ear in cases of earache, ringing in the ear, and deafness.

PAPAYA/Papaya (*Carica papaya*). Papaya is common to the tropics and certainly very much a part of the diets and systems of folk medicine found throughout Latin America. Hispanic immigrants from there find papaya readily available in the warmer-climate states of America, ranging from lower California and stretching all the way eastward to Florida, along the bottom southern half of the country.

Practically everyone with whom I spoke had his or her own favorite remedies involving papaya. Slices of overripe fruit are frequently placed on wounds and open sores to draw out purulent matter and expedite healing. The crushed-green fruit is applied externally as a poultice in cases of severe throat inflammation. A slice of the green fruit is put on ringworm to eradicate it. A decoction of the green, unripe fruit is taken to reduce elevated blood pressure. A small glass of papaya juice is taken to reduce elevated blood pressure. A small glass of papaya juice is taken with a meal in cases of hiatal hernia to prevent food regurgitation later on. Some Cuban-Americans scoop the flesh of the green fruit out, mix it with melted candle wax and coconut oil, and put it back into the papaya skin, which is then placed on hot ashes for 30 minutes. Then the contents are drunk to relieve a cold, flu, or " walking pneumonia." The seeds are often chewed to assist digestion. Puerto Rican folk healers will make an incision in the stem of the palmlike plant, collect the latex that oozes therefrom, and then apply it externally to ringworm, regular warts, plantar's warts, calluses, corns, bunions, and herpes sores to help them clear up. The leaves are made into a cool decoction and used to bathe the skin in cases of erysipelas. The root is crushed and poulticed on the stings of scorpions and jellyfish and on spider bites with good success.

In modern pharmacy, papain, a chief constituent of papaya and a remarkable enzyme, is used in making digestive aids and in preparations to control edema and inflammation associated with surgical or accidental trauma, infections, or allergies. It is also used in certain face creams, cleansers, "face lift" formulations, and dentrifices, and as the active ingredient in enzyme cleansers for soft lenses, among others. Chymopapain, an important secondary constituent of papaya, is very similar to papain in its proteolytic activities and its behavior toward activating and inhibiting agents. The latter is used in the medical treatment of degenerative intervertabral disk disorders (low back pain, sciatica, etc.). Both constituents account for the many remarkable successes claimed for papaya by numerous Hispanic folk healers throughout the Americas.

POLEO/Pennyroyal. This strongly aromatic herb has wonderful applications in any type of pulmonary disorder (pleurisy, asthma, bronchitis, pneumonia, "walking pneumonia," chest cold, influenza, etc.). A *warm* decoction of the leaves and flowers is sweetened with sugar and given to the patient to drink in ½ cup doses every couple of hours; often, *malva* (mallow) and *mentha* (mint) are mixed in with the pennyroyal to make a stronger tea. The other part of this extraordinary folk medical treatment involves—are you ready for this?—pigeons, month-old chicks, and *cucarachos* (cockroaches). The pigeon is cut open and used as a poultice on the chest, and the month-old chick is used, along with prayer, as a *barrida* (magical sweeping) to draw out the illness. The method of preparing the *cucarachos* (cockroaches) is by roasting and crushing, but as to exactly *where* this insect powder is then *inserted*, I'd rather not say out of respect for those who may be somewhat hypersensitive to what may be considered a disgusting practice (but viewed as perfectly normal in *curandismo*). This singular remedy for treating all forms of pulmonary conditions is a classic example of many of the *remedios* so common to Hispanic folk medicine in the United States and elsewhere in Latin America. For here you have a blend of rational medicine and superstition working side by side in perfect harmony. And while the herbal portion is certainly very appealing *and effective* for non-Hispanic users, yet the rest of it won't be for obvious reasons.

HILO ROJO/Red thread. Here is another fine example of Hispanic folk medicine in which superstition prevails entirely over rational medicine; but "cures" are still claimed because of the primitive faith exercised in the practice itself. Red thread is tied around the throat for hiccups or around the big toe for athlete's foot.

SAL/Salt. Jean de Marcounille spoke about what he termed "the sacredness and dignity of salt," in a treatise he wrote on the subject in Paris in 1584. Referring to it as "a mineral," he claimed it "is like unto the four [basic] elements [of life]—earth, air, fire, and water. So universal, so necessary to existence, it is the *fifth element* [of life]." In Hispanic *curanderismo,* salt is frequently employed, often in association with the image of a crucifix. In fact, so high does it rank in terms of domestic importance that it has been referred to at times by different Hispanics as *servicio para el hogar* (a "servant in the house"). Salt water (½ teaspoon of sea salt in 6 ounces of water) makes an effective gargle for sore throat, cleanser of open wounds and runny sores, a mouth wash for halitosis or bad breath, a superb laxative on an empty stomach to relieve constipation, and a dentifrice for sore gums. Folk healers in Hispanic *barrios* throughout the United States rub damp salt on burns, insect stings, itching skin, rashes, or hives to draw out the soreness, though such treatments smart like the devil for a short time. Salt (in this case 1 cup of Epsom salts) added to bath water gives the same effects as a dip in the ocean would: it relieves stress, invigorates a tired body, and soothes jangled nerves. The same salt water makes a comforting bath for tired and aching feet. A simple, safe, and inexpensive body deodorant is salt water applied to the skin wherever odor is likely to occur the most (underarms, groin area, feet) by means of a spray bottle.

But salt is more than a *remedio casero*—it also serves a number of other nonmedical uses as well in Hispanic cultures. A little salt added to parsley makes it chop more easily. Mix 1 heaping pint of salt, a scant pint of lime, and six quarts of water to make an excellent medium in which to store eggs when refrigeration isn't available. Carpet stains may be removed by rubbing them briskly with ordinary table salt; several applications may be necessary, however. Blood stains on cloth vanish when soaked in salt water, washed in warm water with plenty of soap, and then boiled on a hot stove. Salt removes underarm perspiration stains from shirts and blouses.

By sprinkling fine salt over the floors and shelves of your kitchen, indoor ants will soon disappear. Adding a pinch of salt to water in a flower base makes the blooms and leaves remain fresh for a longer time. Sprinkle salt on the crevices of brick and cement walks to kill off weeds and grass. Putting salt at the roots and stalk bases of noxious and nonmedicinal weeds in the yard will kill them; this even includes poison ivy! A good dry cleaner may be had by mixing equal parts of salt and cornmeal moistened with turpentine. Fabric colors won't run in a washing machine when salt is added to the water. Hispanic women who still use flat irons rub them with wax and then scour them with salt when the bottoms get rusty. Rubbing the hands in salt removes the smell of gasoline.

Methods of Application

In Chapter 4, detailed instructions were given for making the different types of natural preparations mentioned in the preceding chapter which extensively covered many ethnobotanical remedies of early Black Americans. Some of the same basic information is given here, but in a slightly different form since the culture (Hispanic) to which this data rightfully belongs is, by itself, distinct from that of blacks.

Practitioners of *curanderismo* utilize herbs mostly in one of three ways: infusion, decoction, or poultice. When fresh herbs are to be made into a medicinal tea of some kind, the folk healer will generally first bruise them by rubbing them between the hands or sometimes using a mortar and pestle to break up the tissue structure and release the active principles. Herbs are often prepared in nonmetallic pots.

Infusion. If a *curandero* or *curandera* is attempting to utilize the volatile oils in herbs such as the mints or the delicate plant parts such as flowers and soft leaves, the herbs are usually steeped in a tightly covered container with water that has just been brought to a rolling boil. This method is called an infusion. The herbs are not boiled at all, as a rule, but are only steeped, allowing 15 to 25 minutes in a tightly covered vessel. I've known some folk practitioners to make a "sun tea" by exposing the herbs in water in a glass fruit jar with the lid screwed on tight in the sun for several hours. And a number of them will also utter short prayers over them, invoking the blessings of different Catholic saints. (The same ritual holds true for decoctions as well.)

Decoction. To extract the deeper essences from coarser leaves, stems, barks, and roots, the herbs are simmered for about an hour. This method is called a decoction. In many cases, the herbs are simmered uncovered and the volume of water is decreased by about half through evaporation. However, some of these coarser herbs contain important volatile oils, and these must be gently simmered or steeped in a covered pot (this mostly applies to roots and barks).

Combining infusion and decoction. There have been a number of occasions where a folk healer will combine roots and barks along with soft leaves and flowers. To make a tea, a decoction is made first with the coarser materials, then strained and poured over the delicate plant parts. This is then steeped, tightly covered, for 15 to 25 minutes, as an infusion usually is.

Poultice. A poultice is a warm, moist mass of powdered or macerated herbs that is applied directly to the skin to relieve inflammation, blood poisoning, venomous bites, and eruptions and to promote proper cleansing and healing of the affected area. Hispanic folk healers believe that poultices have the ability to draw out infection, toxins, and foreign matter embedded within the skin. Poultices are also employed to relieve pain and muscle spasms. It is common in the practice of *curandismo* to give patients a small amount of an herbal stimulant, such as powdered cayenne pepper or ginger root, prior to the application of poultices; these herbs promote strong blood circulation, which is important in the success of poulticing. If powdered herbs are to be used, they are first moistened with hot water, herbal tea, a liniment, or a tincture. Herbs that aren't in powdered form are added by using one of the other extraction methods and then adding them to the powder. I've seen some folk healers use a witch hazel extract, obtained from any drugstore, which is useful for this purpose. And it isn't at all uncommon in the wilds to find a *curandero* or *curandera* who will make a poultice right on the spot by chewing the fresh herbs he or she intends using, before applying them to the affected area.

Finally, something should be said with regard to the almost religious devotion that many Hispanic folk healers approach the practice of *curanderismo*. The really good ones are usually those who employ prayer at different intervals before, during, and after the treatment process, and carry about them what I would describe as a *reverential attitude* while servicing the sick and needy.

This is certainly an inspiring quality which can only benefit patients, for their own hope and faith in the treatment as well as the practitioners are substantially increased when a strong "reverence for life" and deity is genuinely displayed. *True* folk healers are also *more* concerned with the initial welfare of their patients than their economic abilities to pay their modest fees. These qualities separate the hucksters from the healers every time, which is how it should be anyway.

Chapter Nine

FOLK REMEDIES FROM THE UNITED NATIONS

AN A-TO-Z APPROACH TO MAJOR HEALTH PROBLEMS

(ASIA: Afghanistan, Pakistan, Thailand, Indonesia, Philippines, Korea, Vietnam, Japan, China, and Tibet; EUROPE: Great Britain, France, Germany, Italy, Poland, Russia, Spain, and Scandinavia; MIDDLE EAST: Iran, Iraq, Israel, Jordan, Saudi Arabia, and Turkey; POLYNESIA: Hawaii, Samoa, Tonga, Fiji, Tahiti, and New Zealand)

A Global Approach to Folk Medicine

The United Nations (UN) was officially organized on October 24, 1945 (celebrated annually ever since as "UN Day"). The first and only General Assembly meeting to be held on European soil was in London on January 10, 1946; thereafter, the decision was wisely made to locate the UN headquarters somewhere in the Eastern United States. In December 1946, the General Assembly accepted the $8.5 million gift of John D. Rockefeller, Jr., to buy a tract of land along the East River in New York City for its headquarters. The principal buildings there, the Secretariat, the General Assembly, and the Conference Building, were completed in 1952. The Dag Hammaskjöld Memorial Library was dedicated in 1961.

The UN Charter calls for principal organs such as the General Assembly, the Security Council, the Economic and Social Council, the Secretariat, and a few more to administer the organization's main business throughout the world. The Charter, in fact, delineated very clearly the chief purposes for which the UN was formed: (1) to maintain international peace and security; (2) develop friendly relations between various foreign powers; (3) achieve cooperation in solving global economic, social, cultural, and humanitarian problems; and (4) strive for the equality of all men and the expansion of basic freedoms for everyone.

There are, however, a number of other bodies within the framework of the UN that function as specialized agencies but aren't specifically provided for in the Charter itself. These include some well-known ones such as UNESCO (the United Nations Educational, Scientific, and Cultural Organization), headquartered in Paris; UNICEF (United Nations Children's Fund); IMF (the International Monetary Fund), headquartered in Washington, D.C.; and WHO (the World Health Organization), headquartered in Geneva, Switzerland.

UNESCO seeks to further world peace by encouraging a free interchange of ideas and of cultural and scientific achievements, and improving education. A most important long-range UNESCO program concerns the problem of "fundamental education"—teaching people to read and write and to meet the problems of their environment. UNICEF is concerned with assisting children and adolescents throughout the world, particularly in devastated areas and developing countries. The IMF, using a fund of some $28 billion subscribed by the member nations, purchases foreign currencies on application from its members so as to discharge international indebtedness and stabilize exchange rates.

It is with the last of these functioning bodies outside of the UN Charter which we are the most concerned with here. WHO was established in 1948 and admits all sovereign states (including those countries not belonging to the UN) to full membership, as well as admitting territories that are not self-governing to associate membership.

As its very name implies, WHO was formed with a single purpose in mind—to provide "health for all by the year 2000." In carrying out this praiseworthy strategy, it took a novel approach that no one had ever thought of before utilizing *both* conventional as well as folk medical systems in over 100 nations on earth to help prevent the spread of disease, to treat existing health problems, to bolster public nutrition, and to help solve some of the problems of environmental pollution.

The orthodox medical approach to disease containment involved operating public health programs such as sanitation and immunization in over 100 countries. (An almost tragic irony to have developed from the latter course was that in its strident efforts to eradicate small-pox from the planet, WHO somehow ended up using bad batches of live vaccine, which over time may have contributed to the unfortunate development and spread of AIDS.) Providing the basic nutrients such as vitamins A, B, C, and E and minerals like calcium, magnesium, phosphorus, potassium, iron, and iodine through donated supplements to the needy poor of the world, has been of tremendous assistance in maintaining a reasonable measure of "preventive health" among those who are the most susceptible to diseases, namely the young and the elderly.

But it was with its "changed attitude" toward the indigenous systems of simple medicines practiced by numerous cultures that WHO really elevated folk medicine in general and gave it truly global significance in the course of time. No better evidence of this could be found than in the organization's own publication, *World Health* magazine. Beginning as far back as October 1976, there started appearing every so often in different issues articles by folk healers *about* folk healing.

Take the one entitled "A Traditional Doctor Speaks" by J. O. Mume, an herbalist practicing out of "his own nature cure centre" somewhere in rural Nigeria. Portions of the man's essay are quite insightful. "Traditional [folk] medicine has effected wonderful cures with herbs and without the use of well-advertized miracle drugs, surgery or radiation.

"We who carry out this kind of work know that the practice of traditional [folk] medicine is not child's play. We have hundreds of herbal preparations and hundreds of patients, as the years go by. Those who request our aid are in a special class; for them, traditional [folk] medicine has a meaning, even if they do not understand the principles. They do not put themselves in our care just because we are doctors. Perhaps friends have encouraged them, or they may have learnt of some difficult case where the other kind of doctors failed and we have been successful.

"As a single example, take the case of a patient who consulted me. He had been involved in a serious motor accident and had been told by a medical doctor working in a general hospital that one of his legs must be amputated. The patient refused and he was asked to sign a paper conceding the responsibility if the wound resulted in his death. He signed it and determined to consult a tradomedical bone-setter [instead]. I treated the leg with traditional herbal medicines after setting the bones in their proper position. In three weeks the patient started to walk again."

Folk healer Mume concluded his insightful piece this way: "What is clear today is that traditional [folk] medicine has begun to attract so much international attention that the time is ripe for a scientific enquiry into its efficacy. . . . What ought to exist between the two forms of medicine is not hostility but communication and mutual cooperation in order to find answers to diverse human ailments. There is a great need for forums to be sponsored where enlightened herbalists and traditional doctors can exchange views and ideas with 'orthodox' physicians, so that each may learn to respect the other's point of view. . . . [This way] traditional medicine may yet attain new heights and [achieve] greater recognition."

Through its widely circulated publication, WHO has successfully managed to provide a continued forum for folk healers and those who study folk medicine from a scientific perspective, to air their views publicly. Those who practice traditional medicine are of the firm belief that an entire herb ought to be used instead of just its standardized, extracted, active components, as is so popular right now in the commercial herbal medicines currently marketed in many North American health food stores and herb shops. Dr. Chou Chien-Chung, formerly a practitioner of traditional Chinese medicine in the Hsi Yuan Hospital in mainland China, and Dr. Giuseppe Penso, formerly with WHO's Division of Prophylactic, Diagnostic and Therapeutic Substances, teamed up some years ago to contribute to an article in the July 1978 issue of *World Health* magazine entitled, appropriately enough, "Back to Nature."

They gave their logical reasons for being staunch advocates of utilizing the *whole* herb when treating patients. "The action of a medicinal plant results from a small number of specific properties developed by the plant and generally known as the active principles. Besides these, there are certain amounts of other pharmacologically inactive or inert matter, called the vegetable principles.

"Very often these vegetable principles act in conjunction with the active principles, enhancing their therapeutic effects. For example, after the tannins in *Potentilla erecta* [tormentilla cinquefoil] had been isolated, it was thought that, once they had been purified, they might replace the usual drug, powdered *Potentilla* root. But subsequent tests showed that these pure tannins were too strong and that the natural drug gave better relief from diarrhoea since it released the tannins into the digestive tract only gradually, producing a less drastic but more positive effect. Many such examples could be given."

When WHO actually started taking its life-long mission more seriously in 1975 "to provide health for all by the year 2000," its whole position on folk medicine changed dramatically for the better. Between its founding in 1948 and the watershed year of 1975, the orthodox healthcare professionals who managed this organization viewed traditional healing with the same bias and suspicion that most regular doctors everywhere else in the world did.

But then the director-general of WHO at that time, Dr. Halfdan Mahler, made what was then considered to be a radical move on the part of his colleagues by proposing that the very systems of primitive medicine then being practiced by numerous cultures, be "adopted" into the organization's overall healthcare plans along with more conventional medicine. This elevated status gave folk medicine new respectability in the eyes of scientists and healthcare professionals in general.

As Dr. Mahler wrote in an insightful editorial, "The Staff of Aesculapias," in the November 1977 issue of *World Health* magazine: ". . . We in WHO [have] pledged ourselves to an ambitious target: to provide health for all by the year 2000. This ambitious goal is, quite simply, beyond the scope of the present health care system and personnel trained in modern medicine. With so little time left . . . it is clear now that unorthodox solutions must be sought.

"The training of . . . traditional healers may seem very disagreeable to some policy makers, but if the solution is the right one to help people, we should have the courage to insist that this is the best policy in the long run, and is by no means an expedient acceptance of an inferior solution. This is why I have proposed that the great numbers of traditional healers who practice today in virtually every country of the world should not be overlooked.

"The age-old arts of the herbalists must definitely be tapped. Many of the plants familiar to the 'wise-woman' or the 'witch-doctor' really do have the healing powers that tradition attaches to them. The pharmacopoeia of modern medicine would be poorer if one removed from it all the preparations, chemicals, and compounds whose origins lie in herbs, funguses, flowers, fruits, and roots.

"Let us not be in any doubt about this: modern medicine still has a great deal to learn from the collector of herbs and the traditional folk healer. Already I've contacted a number of Ministries of Health, in the developing countries especially, to encourage them to carefully analyze the potions and decoctions used by such traditional healers to determine whether their active ingredients have healing powers that 'science' has somehow overlooked. Whatever the outcome of such scientific testing may be, there is no doubt that the judicious use of such herbs, flowers and other plants for palliative purposes in primary health care can make a major contribution towards reducing a developing country's drug bill. . . . Given goodwill on both sides, such an army of folk healers, traditional birth attendants and herbalists can help to make our goal of health care for all by the year 2000 attainable at last!"

UN Support for Traditional Healing

All administrative functions of the United Nations in New York City are handled by the Secretariat, with the secretary general at its head; the specialized agency of WHO also has a secretariat headed by a director general, but his authority ultimately comes from the proper head of the UN itself.

Since its inception in 1946, the UN has elected seven different secretaries-general. A little bit about them and how they collectively influenced the eventual change in attitudes toward folk medicine may be of corresponding interest to the focus of this chapter.

Trygve Halvdan Lie, a native of Oslo, Norway, was the first UN secretary-general, who served from 1946 to 1953. Although very conservative in his views about many things, he, nonetheless, came in contact with African traditional healing methods in 1959, after quitting his UN post, and being appointed by the General Assembly to mediate a border dispute between Ethiopia and Italy. During time spent in Addis Abba, the capital, he became ill and was subsequently treated by an Ethiopian "wise-woman," who obtained much of her medical information for treating different patients through divination. Yet, he fully recovered and thereafter worked hard with some of his former UN colleagues to have such primitive medicine recognized as a legitimate form of healing.

After him came Dag Hammarskjöld of Sweden, who served from 1953 until September 18, 1961, when he met his death in a plane accident while on a peace mission in the Congo; the plane crashed in Northern Rhodesia (now Zambia). He was one of the most popular and well liked of all the secretaries-general that the UN has ever had and had been reelected unanimously for another term of five years in September 1957. He worked diligently to prevent war in the Middle East during the Suez Canal crisis.

His acquaintance with folk medicine came about in a rather unusual way. He went on a vital diplomatic peace mission to Beijing, China, from December 30, 1954, to January 13, 1955, in order to obtain the release of 15 detained American fliers who had served under the UN Command in Korea. While there, he learned that one of the pilots had become seriously ill with hepatitis, but had fully recovered under the kind care of some "barefoot doctors" who practiced a combination of traditional Chinese herbal medicine and classical acupuncture on him. The secretary-general became intrigued enough with this type of folk medicine that he strongly encouraged healthcare professionals at WHO in Geneva to start investigating the merits of such treatments. His untimely death, however, prevented a followthrough on such a wise suggestion. Prejudice and ignorance among medical personnel at WHO headquarters caused a quick and silent death of any further research into Chinese traditional medicine for at least another decade or so.

The third secretary-general of the UN was U Thant of Myanmar (formerly known as Burma). He served from 1961 to 1971. Prior to his appointment as permanent representative of Burma to the United Nations (1957–1961), he was a freelance journalist, broadcaster, and high school teacher. He contributed several articles to Rangoon newspapers on Burmese village medicine that were both favorable and encouraging. When he was chosen to head the world body of the UN following Hammarskjöld's tragic demise, he used the power of his office to artfully persuade WHO personnel in Switzerland to look more positively at folk healing in general.

His successor, Kurt Waldheim of Austria (1972–1981), a smart lawyer and astute politician, was the one, though, who really put some teeth into his constant admonitions with WHO personnel that they fairly evaluate folk medicine on its own merits and without their usual prejudices. What prompted this was a small, unforeseen incident which occurred in February 1973 when Waldheim made an official trip to the Indian subcontinent. His chief purpose in being there was to discuss with the governments of India, Pakistan, and Bangladesh, the problems created by the border war between India and Pakistan and find hopeful solutions to overcome its devastating consequences.

One of the translators who had accompanied him there, a fellow European and close friend who spoke fluent Hindi, became unexpectedly ill due to drinking some bad water. The man was treated by skilled Ayurvedic doctors using the food spice turmeric, which is wonderful for liver ailments such as hepatitis. Waldheim was so impressed with his aide's recovery that, upon his return to New York City, he undertook decisive steps to ensure that WHO personnel in Geneva would "get the message" to consider using folk healers as part of their global healthcare initiative.

A Peruvian by the name of Javier Perez De Cuellar assumed office as the fifth secretary-general of the UN on January 1, 1982, and served until the end of December 1991. Prior to his appointment as

permanent representative of his country to the UN, he served as am-
bassador of Peru, first to Switzerland, then the former Soviet Union,
followed by Poland, and finishing up with Venezuela. This now retired lawyer and diplomat has been decorated by some 25 different
countries during the course of his lengthy career.

His grandmother achieved some minor renown in Lima as a practicing *curandera,* and this carried over to his mother, though to a
much lesser extent. While his influence in the promulgation of folk
medicine may not have been felt as directly with officials at WHO,
his quiet and behind-the-scenes efforts in this direction were no less
supportive than those of his predecessors.

Under the indirect leadership of the UN's sixth secretary-general,
an Egyptian lawyer-scholar-diplomat named Boutros Boutros-Ghali
(1992–1996), the World Health Organization continued its basic education programs with folk healers throughout the world in teaching
them hygiene, nutrition, and simple medical procedures for emer-
gency situations (CPR, first aid, etc.). His term, however, was one of
the shortest on account of his sometimes confrontational style and
fractious personality.

The current and seventh secretary-general, Kofi Annan, is from
Ghana and began serving on January 1, 1997. In June 2000 he was
elected to a second five-year term. With degrees in economics and
management, he began a systematic study of the most cost-effective
way of dealing with the worldwide HIV/AIDS epidemic in conjunction with WHO. Under his inspiring guidance, the decision was made
to more actively solicit the assistance of folk healers in different nations and to use their collective wisdom in dealing with this global
health catastrophe.

Thus, we can see for the most part that there has always been
some type of support for traditional healing at the United Nations
from those men who've served as its secretary-general. With some
the endorsement has been rather unobtrusive, while with others it
was more aggressive and very apparent. Yet their combined efforts
put the WHO on a path and in a direction from which it would never
turn back nor regret. And because of this, folk medicine in all of its
many diverse forms has achieved international respectability with

many, many people, including some of its former, fiercest, medical opponents.

Natural Remedies for Twenty Health Problems

In the course of my extensive fieldwork with folk medicine in the last three decades, I've had several opportunities through the auspices of UN's World Health Organization to make contact with traditional healers from a number of different countries. With a few exceptions, most of them were willing to participate in my research and permit me to work alongside them, quietly observing, taking notes, and sometimes asking questions where appropriate as they treated their many patients.

The valuable data gleaned from this on-site and hands-on investigative work has been collated and applied to the TOP TWENTY health problems which the World Health Organization and its parent agency the United Nations consider to be the most important ailments afflicting humanity right now. They are listed below in alphabetical order:

THE WORLD'S TOP TWENTY HEALTH PROBLEMS

1. AIDS	11. Fever
2. Addiction	12. Heart disease
3. Allergy	13. Hepatitis
4. Arthritis	14. Hypertension
5. Asthma	15. Mental illness
6. Cancer	16. Obesity
7. Constipation	17. Sexually transmitted diseases
8. Depression	18. Tuberculosis
9. Diabetes	19. Underweight
10. Diarrhea	20. Worms

AIDS. Acquired immune deficiency syndrome has now become the world's biggest health threat. This horrible and devastating disease is now found on every continent of the earth, and cases have been officially confirmed in 141 of the 186 countries listed with the UN.

Many different approaches to its treatment have been tried, both orthodox as well as nonconventional. Some have had limited measures of success, while others have proven to be of no lasting value. In their efforts to deal with this deadly problem in their own way, the Japanese, Chinese, Tibetans, Vietnamese, Thais, and Koreans have come up with a relatively simple solution that is both safe and inexpensive and seems to be getting worthwhile results.

It is maitake *(Grifolia frondosa),* an edible mushroom that grows in clusters on hardwood trees throughout much of the Northern Hemisphere. Mushroom experts believe the rippling shape of the fungus earned it the Japanese name *maitake,* which means "dancing mushroom."

Americans, Europeans, and Southeast Asians now cultivate it as a gourmet mushroom. Rich in vitamin D, maitake is said to taste like roasted chicken.

The initial research into maitake began with the Japanese some years ago, but eventually expanded into other countries of Southeast Asia, such as China, Thailand, and Korea, where scientists soon discovered its incredible immune-enhancing powers. The collective data from all of this Asian research has shown that what makes maitake work so well against life-threatening infections like AIDS is its polysaccharides; these naturally occurring plant sugars contain beta glucans which stimulate the human immune system in an amazing way. This offers protection not only against AIDS and other existing forms of cancer, but also severely *limits* their spread in existing cases. Beta glucans have been shown to enhance immune functions in those already infected with HIV.

Most of the published studies on maitake have been in test tubes or on animals, but a few fairly recent reports have included human trials as well. A lab study published in 2000 in an issue of *Molecular Urology* found that maitake fought cancer almost unbelievably well. A liquid extract of maitake beta glucans killed more than 95 percent of prostate cancer cells in a test tube within 24 hours.

Two Japanese studies done on mice in the late 1980s found that maitake extract substantially increased the power of killer T-cells and macrophages, two very important elements of the immune system. Maitake's ability to boost the immune system in ways that no other natural substance seems capable of doing has led a number of doctors throughout Southeast Asia to begin prescribing it to many of their HIV or AIDS cases, with apparently very good results.

Maitake is available fresh or dried for cooking and as a supplement in powder, pill, and liquid forms. A recommended daily intake for general health enhancement is somewhere between 3 to 5 grams of the power or capsules. For liquid extracts, between 15 to 30 drops three times daily is advised. A month's supply of maitake for medicinal purposes will generally run somewhere around $30. (See the Appendix for a reliable source of this highly efficient natural treatment for HIV and AIDS.)

There are obviously many different approaches to the treatment and control of AIDS. Some involve lifestyle adjustments; others require dietary changes; and a lot of others employ a variety of substances, some natural and some unnatural. But from what the current evidence has thus far demonstrated, it is fair to say that maitake mushroom has emerged as the world leader in the treatment and control of a vicious disease that claims hundreds of thousands of victims every year with no end in sight.

ADDICTION.   Addiction is a worldwide problem affecting an estimated one billion people in one form or another. The most common addictions include alcohol, cocaine, heroin, marijuana, nicotine, caffeine, eating disorders, sex, and gambling. Most of them are health-destroying in some way, but all of them are quite expensive.

It has become increasingly more difficult for many addicts to simply walk away from their vices and resist the temptation to fondly look back for a later get-together with them. But *anything* is possible if there is willpower, determination, and patience. A combination of four things has proven to be the most successful for permanently disavowing one's bad vices.

They include detoxification, chiropractic, acupuncture, and supplementation. The initial detox phase has long been a fixture of Greek and Islamic folk medicines. Chiropractic is very much an American invention that has taken hold in Canada, Great Britain, and other parts of Europe. Acupuncture originated with the Chinese and still remains one of their healing fortés, although it is now practiced elsewhere in the world by healthcare providers from other cultures. Supplementation is again more of an American thing, although it has been catching on in places like Russia and Japan.

Detoxification has always been a primary consideration in Greece and Islamic countries such as Iran, Iraq, Jordan, Saudi Arabia, and Turkey. In these places the idea of assisting the body in throwing off addictive substances which have been ingested is an old and established idea.

Methods of detoxing will vary, of course, depending on which country or culture you're in at the time. Sweating through the inducement of hot steam baths or saunas is pretty much common to all of those previously cited. A mild food fast is found in a few of them but not in all.

Here is a brief synopsis of how the Greeks and Turks do it. The first four days of the mild food diet consists of all the legumes, fruits, nuts, seeds, vegetables, and whole grains that a recovering addict wishes to have. Some of these aforementioned cultures will include a tonic drink consisting of water mixed with lemon juice to cleanse the liver, honey or dates and figs for nourishment, ginger root tea to relieve nausea, and mints to aid digestion and improve blood circulation.

After staying on this regimen for four days, the recovering addict now enters a two-day fruit and vegetable fast in which he or she is allowed to eat any fruits and vegetables of his or her choosing—but only these and *nothing else!* Sometimes turmeric root for liver and gallbladder stimulation and psyllium seed or figs for colon revival may be added, but not in every case.

After a week's time on such a loosely constructed detox program, the turnaround for most former addicts is truly astonishing. Their cravings have disappeared; they report feeling more stamina and energy; many of their usual allergy symptoms have disappeared by now; and all declare that they're able to get a good night's rest for a change.

Chiropractic is something distinctly American and in the year 2001 celebrated its 103rd year in existence as a primary healthcare alternative. Jay M. Holder, D.C., M.D., Ph.D., who practices out of Miami and Miami Beach, Florida, also directs the 300-bed Exodus Addiction Treatment Center there, which has been a blessing for several thousand addicts.

A fully recovered alcoholic came to see Dr. Holder a few years ago, after suffering from depression, displaying psychotic behavior, and being strung out on alcohol and cocaine at the same time. He'd seen four psychiatrists, who had given him different mood-altering drugs, which only worsened his condition. He had started two addiction programs, but finished neither and attended Alcoholics Anonymous meetings but quit when he found them utterly "boring and useless" (as he put it). He'd go off illicit substances for a few weeks, even a few months, but then experience another relapse.

He came to see Dr. Holder, who examined his spine and found out which particular vertebra was out of alignment. Once the subluxation was correctly identified, he was given a number of weekly physical adjustments spanning the course of several months. Dr. Holder believes that chiropractic is absolutely necessary in reversing addictions. "A subluxation [or out-of-place spinal vertebra] interferes with your body's ability to function in a whole way, which is a form of neurological insult," he claims. "Any addict will have a spine with at least one or more vertebrae out of alignment. This even goes for those with eating disorders and gambling," he insists.

Besides correcting addicts' misalignments, Dr. Holder also starts them on a series of four amino acids, which are precursors or building blocks for the proteins normally found in foods. This daily oral supplementation includes: DL-phenylalanine (750 mg, 3 times), 5-hydroxytryptophan (500 mg, 3 times), L-glutamine (750 mg), and L-tyrosine (500 mg, 3 times). Dr. Holder usually keeps his addict patients on this amino acid combination for at least a year into their recovery.

Specifically, these amino acids, especially DL-phenylalanine, the "addiction-treatment king," will help the brain to restore the "brain reward cascade" and the bodywide sense of well-being it invariably induces. By reducing stress and lifting depression, they will help recovering addicts make important changes in their behavior and attitude, which are crucial to the success of their treatment programs.

In addition to chiropractic and supplementation, there is also acupuncture. Classical Chinese traditional medicine describes five ear points in acupuncture which produce beneficial results. Recent neurological research has shown that there are four important cranial nerves that have nerve endings throughout the ear. Some of the more innovative Oriental acupuncturists will use a microcurrent rather than the customary needles with their addict patients. This form of acupuncture is known as auriculotherapy and greatly relaxes addicts. It also enables them to feel less apathetic and more highly motivated to stay off drugs. It reduces drug cravings and their sense of physical and emotional withdrawal.

Acupuncturists who employ a microcurrent instead of needles use a small hand-held probe that delivers between 5 and 20 Hz in microcurrent to specific ear points for 15 to 30 seconds per point. This compares to needle-delivered ear acupuncture that requires anywhere from 45 to 60 minutes of stimulation in order to get the same results. This microcurrent is painless, efficient, and specific, and assists in the release of pleasure-producing brain chemicals called endorphins more quickly and thoroughly than needle treatment does.

Dr. Holder's average monthly program for treating addictions usually runs somewhere between $1,100 and $1,400, as compared to other programs costing as much as $16,000 a month. He explains addiction this way: "It is compulsive use of a chemical or activity in spite of negative consequences." You keep using a substance even though you know it's bad for you. There are five types of addiction, including work, food, sex, drugs, chemicals, and gambling, and each one has many factors. "But these five categories are all variations of just one disease—addiction!" he claims.

ALLERGY.   This is fairly common around the world in some form or another. It is a state of hypersensitivity induced by exposure to a particular antigen (allergen) resulting in harmful immunologic reactions on subsequent exposures. Spring is usually a bad time for those frequently prone to an allergy of some sort. As the trees bud, the flowers bloom, and the grasses green, a host of new life springs forth: pesky pollens, molds, and other allergens that can wreak havoc on nose, eyes, skin and sinuses.

Although the allergy may lurk all year round, often unnoticed, symptoms generally become more acute in late spring and summer, when the irritating plant is pollinating and blooming or when wet weather spawns the growth of mold. All it takes for a flare-up is the inhalation of small allergen particles. The allergens bind to the antibodies known as immunoglobulin E (or IgE), which attach to cells, causing the cells to produce and release histamines. The histamines, in turn, cause the dilation of small blood vessels—for example, in the nose—sometimes unleashing fluid. The results: runny nose, watery eyes, and itchy skin.

As unbearable as an allergy may be, however, a form of folk medicine that over time has become recognized more as an alternative medicine is homeopathy. It can ease and often eliminate allergy symptoms. I myself have never been a proponent of it and wish to go on record saying that once when I made it a matter of personal prayer, I was answered thusly by Him who knows all things: "John, this is *not* a system of medicine ordained by me!" That and nothing more.

However, I am wise enough to realize that it does work for many people and, therefore, feel an obligation to include it here. Based on the principle that "like cures like" (known as the law of similars), homeopathic remedies consist of highly diluted amounts of plant, mineral, and animal substances that can actually ease the symptoms a patient suffers from. Homeopathic doctors give their patients a little dose of something that mimics the allergy symptoms they have. Often that causes a temporary flare-up followed by an immediate improvement.

Typical allergy symptoms are an autoimmune response to allergens, and homeopathy reportedly strengthens the immune system, thereby increasing the body's ability to ward off disease. By intensifying the symptoms, so the thinking goes, homeopathy signals the body's defense mechanisms to overcome the illness.

Conventional allergy medicines such as antihistamines, on the other hand, suppress symptoms and can cause side effects like sleepiness and headaches. But these medicines don't aid in healing the body as homeopathics do. With homeopathy, advocates declare, the individual and his or her symptoms are looked at and the symptoms themselves then treated accordingly. Instead of trying to suppress the body's reaction to something, homeopathics strengthens the person's vitality.

It is always best to work with a professional homeopath instead of going it alone with homeopathic remedies that can be easily purchased from most health food stores. (In Europe, India, and Mexico, such homeopathics are generally obtained from a licensed homeopathic pharmacy or apothecary or homeopathic doctor rather than from a health food store or herb shop.)

The World Health Organization has been in favor of homeopathy for a long time. Those who practice it in their native lands to quell the coughing, itchy throat, runny nose, or watery eyes that typically accompany an allergy will rely on these particular remedies:

Allium cepa (onion):   Symptoms mimic those of exposure to onion—profuse runny nose, aggravated by warmth.

Euphrasia (eyebright):   Main characteristic is a burning, watery eye discharge without a lot of nasal discharge.

Nux vomica (poison nut):   Symptoms are marked by sneezing attacks in the morning. At night there's a tendency for the nose to get stuffed up.

Sabadilla (from the lily family):   The main indication for this remedy is violent and prolonged sneezing.

Pulsatilla (windflower):   Thick, bland nasal discharge, lack of thirst, worse in a warm room.

The treatments that homeopathic doctors offer to allergy sufferers is always an individualized process. They always look for the remedy that fits the individual. The trick, of course, is to uncover the pattern of symptoms for each person that will lead to an appropriate remedy.

Symptoms in allergy are observable and easy to discern. The differences in symptoms can be subtle, but important and unique. For instance, the way a person's nose feels, whether it's itchy or not, whether the mucus is thick or runny, what time of day the allergy sufferer feels fatigued, whether the symptoms are worse in a closed room or in an open space. Those are the types of things that homeopathic doctors tune into.

Once a homeopath has this kind of data, he or she prescribes a remedy to match the patient's unique symptoms. All these things come together to create a remedy picture; the remedy resonates with the symptoms, according to homeopathic beliefs.

Often, the end result is that an allergy hits the high road. A French homeopathic doctor recalled one of his best success stories for me a while back. His patient Pierre suffered so badly from an allergy that he could barely function as an artist. At the height of ragweed season, he'd be positively miserable. The thing that was looked at in his particular situation was not just the physical symptoms alone, but his mental and emotional states as well. Such as what kind of grief and level of anxiety he experienced, the types of foods he craved, the forms of relationships he had. All those things came together to create a remedy picture. My French informant chose lycopodium (club moss), which is typically indicated for those with anxiety related to work, as well as headaches, tickling cough, and rattling mucus. As a result, Pierre's allergy improved dramatically—and so did his overall outlook on life.

The French doctor stated that "in its highest form, homeopathy treats the entire person. We see not just the allergy shift, but the person himself shift as well."

Besides homeopathy, which I have never believed in for the prior reason given, there is also a very simple dietary adjustment which, if made, can reduce allergy symptoms by 65 percent or better. This is one I've long put into practice not only with myself but with thousands of others as well and know from personal experience that it works fabulously in defeating *most* symptoms.

It is so simple and yet as difficult for many to diligently apply; but those who do are forever rid of their allergies or at least can manage with what few symptoms may periodically remain. The adjustment is this: Leave sugar alone and avoid *all* sweet things as much as possible. Believe it or not, *it actually works!*

ARTHRITIS. Over a decade ago, separate teams of rheumatologists working independently of each other at the Stanford Arthritis Center in Stanford, California, and the Veterans Hospital in Columbia, Missouri, made a wonderful discovery: rheumatoid arthritis patients who decreased their depression and increased their sense of personal effectiveness were far better at pain control. And *helping others* was the single, powerful key to eradicating most depression and gaining greater self-mastery over seemingly impossible situations.

As Fawriza El-Adnan, a 51-year-old switchboard operator at the United Nations who suffers from rheumatoid arthritis, told me a few years ago, "Ever since I began with older Egyptian immigrants within my neighborhood and community, and helping them in different ways, I've felt a lot better about myself. And strangely enough, since I've been in so much demand with these seniors, assisting them with medical documents or insurance papers they don't understand, I've completely forgotten about the aches and pains of the occasional arthritis which used to trouble me a great deal more."

That helping others can have this kind of relieving power may seem paradoxical, given that coming to the aid of another can bring one face to face with someone else who also has problems that could make the helper feel more inadequate or disappointed. But none of this seems to impair the effect.

Helping should be viewed a lot like exercise: It is the *process* itself that is the healing factor here, without regard to its outcome. It doesn't really matter if a helper is able to solve someone else's problems or experience disappointment if his or her assistance is rejected. It's the health benefits produced by helping others that really count in the long run; they compare favorably with the best results obtained by regular exercise as well as painkilling or mood-elevating medication.

But unlike exercise, helping has a vast potential to benefit the health of not only the individual but also our entire tension-ridden society. According to the results of one study sponsored by the University of Cairo, which involved participants from a local Muslim community there, those volunteers suffering from rheumatoid arthritis who involved themselves in a variety of helping acts experienced not only good feelings but also an immediate reduction in their overall pain. And as their empathy for others—particularly strangers—increased, so, too, did their own personal health. As awareness spreads of the powerful sense of well-being and related health benefits, more people such as these are likely to try to perform helping acts, leading to a new level of daily altruism in society, and in addition, volunteers are helped to better cope with their physical pains without medications.

ASTHMA.   We have the Arabs to thank for the cultural, pleasurable, and medicinal benefits of coffee. Coffee was known to them in the fifteenth century; from there it spread to Egypt and Turkey, overcoming religious and political opposition to become popular with all of the Arab world.

At first proscribed by Italian churchmen as an infidel's drink, it was approved by Pope Clement VIII, and by the midseventeenth century, coffee had reached most of Europe. Introduced in North America around 1668, coffee became a favorite American beverage after the Boston Tea Party made tea unfashionable.

Herodotus (485–425 B.C.), the acknowledged Father of History (as Cicero designated him), mentioned in his extensive history that Arabia was "the only country which yields a dark, bitter beverage that they say is good for diseases of the lungs when taken hot." Once I had made this discovery some years ago for myself, I began recommending the *gradual* sipping of hot, black coffee through a plastic straw (so as not to burn the mouth or tongue) for those suffering from either asthma or bronchitis. The results obtained were almost instantaneous: sufferers reported immediate relief from chest congestion and a greater ability to breathe within minutes after finishing their cups of hot coffee, *sans* milk and sugar.

The coffee seeds (commonly called "cherries") are extremely high in caffeine content (usually 1.5–3.2%) in their green form before being roasted. It is this important alkaloid which acts as a very effective vaso-bronchodilator, in that it reduces constriction of blood vessels in lung muscles and greatly expands the bronchial tubes in both lungs, thereby facilitating the intake of more oxygen into the body through the mechanism of breathing.

CANCER. The Europeans, especially the Germans, French, Italians, Poles, and Spaniards, know something about cancer that we don't—an extract of mistletoe (*Viscum album*) has been the favored remedy of choice among laypeople and doctors alike in treating many forms of cancer with a relatively high success rate.

Mistletoe is a semiparasitic shrub with yellow-green stems and white berries common to Europe and Asia and found on almost all deciduous trees (except for beech); two subspecies occur only on conifers. The definite antitumor activity in mistletoe berry and herb lies in the lectins which parts contain; the polysaccharides that are present also participate in the working of these lectins against cancer.

A number of mistletoe preparations intended for injection purposes only are made by different European pharmaceutical companies; Iscador, Plenosol, and Helixor are three of the most popular brands currently available. Of these, the first has been drawing the most media attention of late, because well-known TV actress Suzanne Somers has opted to use it to treat her breast cancer instead of conventional chemotherapy, cobalt radiation, and surgery. She has been severely criticized by the regular medical establishment for lending support and giving so much hype to something they still consider to be a form of quack medicine. Yet, to all appearances, she seems to be doing just fine and her cancer is in remission as of this writing.

A recent study published in the May 2001 issue of *Alternative Therapies in Health and Medicine* followed more than 10,000 German cancer patients. About one-fifth used Iscador and a conventional treatment; the rest received only conventional care. Researchers concluded that those who took Iscador lived 40 percent longer.

The history behind Iscador is as lively as it is controversial. It began as a simple folk remedy widely utilized by German and Swiss herbalists in the latter part of the nineteenth-century. Anthroposophist Rudolf Steiner, who founded a twentieth century religious system that emphasized the importance of man over God, invented a secret process by which the most active constituents of mistletoe were extracted and then used for cancer therapy; this occurred in 1920 and was eventually tested by the Society for Cancer Research in Arlesheim, Switzerland, which proved its definite efficacy in this area. But because the image of Steiner as sort of a "nut case" lingers in some parts of the world, Iscador is still viewed with considerable prejudice in places like Great Britain, Canada, and the United States in spite of its obvious track record.

CONSTIPATION. In ancient times, *enemas ruled* in such countries as Egypt and India. The Egyptian medical papyri of the time frequently mentioned enemas in association with constipation. Egyptian medical belief took the anus as the center and stronghold of decay; the dreaded *ukhedu* ("rotten stuff par excellence") originated there and could travel via the blood vessels throughout the rest of the body, setting up disease wherever it pleased.

Hence, great efforts were made to keep ruling pharaohs and their royal families free from constipation and the awful *ukhedu*. Inscriptions on the tombs of some of these ancient doctors mentioned the various titles they were given according to their specific professions—"Guardian of the Royal Bowel Movement" meant no less than a physician whose sole duty was to carefully monitor his majesty's bathroom activities and see to it that "things kept moving" along nicely without any obstructions.

The idea for the enema came from Egyptian observation of the ibis, a once sacred bird with a glistening white body and black head, which stood in the water along the banks of the Nile River, and presumably washed its insides out by introducing its long beak into its rectum frequently. In the instructions of the Ebers papyrus is found this oft-repeated sentence, "Let be poured into his rectum." A cattle horn, its sharp end clipped off so as to create a small opening, served the doctors as the instrument for giving enemas, which consisted of such interesting components as ox gall, fats, and extremely potent laxatives like senna, which can really evacuate tightly packed bowels in explosive hurry!

DEPRESSION.   Korean, Chinese, and Filipino immigrants to America have learned how to cope with depression in the same remarkable way that they did in their native lands. This is by forming strong family ties and equally strong neighborhoods. Ever notice how these different ethnic groups prefer hanging out with their own kind? It used to be that way with Italian, German, Polish, and Russian immigrants during the first part of the twentieth century, but that phenomenon gradually waned as the older generations died off and the younger ones moved away from the local neighborhoods in search of lives of their own.

Oriental neighborhoods, however, are still the kind of communities we want to remember but are fast disappearing from the social landscape of our once great nation. In Koreatowns, Chinatowns, or Filipino Barrios, as they are usually called, people still rely upon each other for friendship and assistance. They don't let the hectic schedules of everyday life keep them from establishing such beneficial relationships. Everyone knows their neighbors, sometimes perhaps a little too well.

Because of such tightly knit communities as these, there is very little depression to be found in young or old alike. There is a general sense of caring, and everyone's emotional well-being is helped by each other. Rather than remain isolated and fragmented, they are all a unified part of a whole society, so no one ever feels truly alone as it is with the rest of us.

To get out of the doldrums you're in, begin thinking of ways that you can reconnect again with your community in some way. Begin by researching what you might be able to contribute; the possibilities are endless and the website www.volunteermatch.org is just the place to start. You just enter your zip code and answer a few questions (for example, "How far can you travel?") and the site provides a list of possible activities and contact information.

If formal volunteering seems daunting, think of other ways you can help your community. Perhaps you could get up early one morning and pick up trash in the neighborhood. Or maybe there's an elderly person nearby with whom you could visit one afternoon. Do you know an overwhelmed parent? Offer to babysit for free one evening. How about serving as a volunteer in a school reading program somewhere for children who are slow learners? Or offering to drive sight-impaired individuals to the supermarket, doctor, church, or anywhere else they may need to go.

The point is that you lose yourself in the service of others, and soon the things that caused your despondency pretty much clear up of their own accord, so long as you remain busily engaged in community affairs of some kind.

Folk healers in Hawaii known as *kahunas* often turn to *limu* or seaweed to help their patients overcome depression. *Limu* is usually eaten raw, and dressed or sauced with coconut cream (which is expressed from grated coconut) or fresh coconut out of the shell that's been grated. The same holds true also when one examines the folk remedies for depression in Tonga, Tahiti, Fiji, and Samoa. Since seaweeds are naturally high in iodine (good for the thyroid) and numerous trace elements (good for the body's "master glands" like pineal, pituitary, and thymus), they are capable of giving a powerful nutritional boost to human systems that are in short supply of these vital nutrients and subsequently in states of mental and emotional depressions as a rule. I've never met anyone yet who frequently subsisted on seaweeds who was ever depressed; and *that's a fact!*

The other alternative, for those lacking a taste for seaweeds and algaes, is nutritional supplementation, of course. Two companies stand out among many in terms of what they offer and how effective such quality products can be. Naturally Vitamins of Phoenix, Arizona, sells Valerian Super Stress (Valerian, B vitamins, and other calming herbs), Primrose Gold (evening primrose oil), and Lipomega 6 (borage seed oil), which a number of naturopathic doctors find helpful for getting their patients out of the blues. Then there is Earth's Pharmacy out of Farmington, Utah, which markets through mail order SAMe (s-adenosylmethionine), B-Well, and St. John's wort, which form another core program of equal value in the nutritional battle against depression. Consumers are advised to follow the suggested daily intakes indicated for all of these products as found on their respective labels. (See the back Appendix for additional information on where to obtain them.)

(Readers may wish to check under MENTAL ILLNESS in this section for additional nutritional data.)

DIABETES. My grandmother Barbara Kaplan Liebhardt Heinerman was born and grew up in Temesvar, Hungary (now Timisoara, Rumania). As a young child, I listened with fascination to the many wonderful healing stories she told, as well as watched with considerable interest as she treated people with folk remedies. I shall never forget the day when I, as a five-year-old, asked her "Grandma, why do so many people come to you?" Nor will I forget the classic answer she gave in return: "John, it is because they have usually had a frustrating experience with a regular medical doctor and come to see someone like your grandma to make them better." Here it was, plain as the nose on your face: a university-educated medical doctor with lettered degrees behind the name versus a village peasant with limited education and no degrees but confident in the folk medical wisdom and healing gift which God endowed this simple soul with.

Grandmother remembered what it was like in nineteenth-century Hungary and left behind a record in her native German of such things, which I have translated into English. "In the Szatmár region [Transylvania], the Hungarian peasants possessed considerable forests or clusters of sweet chestnut trees, without having to care for them. The chestnuts were regularly gathered in autumn, and eaten roasted or boiled.

"Anybody was free to gather the fruit of privately owned chestnut trees after All-Saints' Day [November 1]. This was when I would gather quantities of these fruits to make into strong tea or a mush. I would give one or the other [or sometimes both] to people suffering from blood sugar problems [such as diabetes and hypoglycemia]. This was a very good remedy in those times for such things.

"Special implements were used for the gathering, such as wooden tweezers for picking up the chestnuts in their thorny husks, wooden hammers for removing the fruits from those husks. Eventually, the chestnuts were trampled out of their thorny green husks by myself or my husband [Jacob Heinerman, Sr.]; we would wear top boots for this purpose. A wooden rake and a special kind of implement—called a *kocsorba* in Hungarian—were used to gather the ripened chestnuts. The chestnuts would be roasted in an iron pan. The consumption of sweet chestnuts is something I still miss from the old country."

DIARRHEA.   An effective Tibetan remedy to stop the "runs" calls for 10 parts sweet almonds and 1 part bitter almonds (apricot pits) to be soaked in water with an equal amount of white rice; the water should cover these food materials by several inches. After the almonds and rice are well soaked and become tender, they should be ground into a paste using a mortar and pestle or small food mill of some kind. The resulting milky mixture is strained to remove the coarse particles, and then diluted with a little water and cooked with some sugar to improve the flavor. The finished liquid has a consistency ranging from soupy thin to gruel thick, depending on the amount of water or rice used.

This drink is taken frequently throughout the day, 1 or 2 cups at a time. The active principles (amygdalin or laetrile) in the almonds, which contain traces of natural cyanide, will kill off whatever intestinal bacteria are present that are causing the diarrhea, while the heavy starch from the white rice will tend to tighten the stool. Generally, after 1 to 2 days' treatment, the diarrhea will have ceased.

FEVER.   For a number of centuries, feverfew (*Pyrethrum parthenium*) has been the standard choice of many herbalists throughout the British Isles for dispelling any kind of fever. This composite plant grows in nearly every hedgerow there and is adorned with delightful, small, daisylike yellow flowers with outer white rays and central golden florets. The stem is finely furrowed and hairy, about 2 feet high, and the alternate leaves are downy with short hairs, or nearly smooth. Often this plant has been mistaken for wild chamomile. The entire plant has a strong and bitter smell and is purposely avoided by honey bees.

In olden times, a few of these freshly picked plants would be bound on the wrists of fever sufferers as a further inducement for its reduction. But it has always been with the strong brew itself that high body temperatures and chills have been cleared up when taken regularly. The feverish body would also be sponged with some of this tea to keep biting insects away, such as annoying mosquitos, nasty gnats, thirsty ticks, and bored bed bugs.

Modern research has shown feverfew to be efficacious for controlling migraine headaches. A 1985 double-blind placebo-governed trial on the use of this herb as a prophylactic treatment for migraine assessed a 25-milligrams dose of freeze-dried leaf capsules on 17 patients, and concluded that, when take prophylactically, the plant reduces the frequency and severity of migraine symptoms. A 1988 randomized, double-blind, placebo-controlled trial involving 72 volunteers clearly associated feverfew treatment with a reduction in the frequency of vomiting commonly associated with migraine attacks as well as a reduction in their overall severity.

HEART DISEASE. Hong Kong herbalists and Chinese herb doctors practicing traditional Chinese medicine in Jakarta, Indonesia, frequently rely on *shan zha* fruit (*Crataegus pinnatifida* or hawthorn berry) and a little bit of *yin guo* seed (Ginko biloba) and red pepper powder to calm a restless heart, dilate the coronary arteries, and increase blood flow, as well as treating angina and mild congestive heart failure.

Forms of administration include a tea or encapsulated or tableted powder. The standard mixture for any of these is always 7 parts hawthorn fruit, 2 parts cayenne pepper, and 1 part ginko biloba. They are recommended to be taken with meals twice daily.

HEPATITIS. This is one of the world's leading diseases, owing to poor sanitation, lack of proper hygiene in food preparation, and bad water. The Ayurvedic doctors of India for many centuries have recommended two basic herbs to combat this potentially fatal disease, turmeric root (in the form of curry powder) and raw garlic bulb.

While it is true that turmeric (*Curcuma longa*) and garlic (*Allium sativa*) may be conveniently taken in capsule forms to mask the unpleasant taste and hide the offensive odor), Indian folk healers insist that these spices should always be used in their *fresh* state and, preferably, in meals. The two used together in curry dishes can correct even the severest cases of hepatitis if given a year to do so. In conjunction with this, hepatitis patients should be encouraged to drink lots of tomato juice or low-sodium V8; tomato juice is terrific for the liver and provides the body with a great deal of energy, believe it or not!

HYPERTENSION.   The French are the biggest consumers of homeopathic products in the world simply because they are convinced that such things work. (But then again, they're equally notorious for taking more medicines of virtually all kinds than anyone else in Europe, including antibiotics, tranquilizers, and antidepressants, while continuing to down the most alcohol and the most miraculous healing water from Lourdes.)

It is said by many Frenchmen (and their women, too) that Charlemagne, Emperor of the West and King of the Franks, ordered fields of medicinal herbs planted in his domains. Whenever he became ill, he would go out into these vast herb gardens, throw his sword into one of them, and let God decide which plant would heal him—by using whatever his weapon was found near. That is how watercress or the mustard-and-cress variety came to be used for high blood pressure. Charlemagne suffered from high blood pressure, but noticed its almost immediate reduction upon consuming platefuls of raw cress.

MENTAL ILLNESS.   The woman came at a trot up the steep valley side, her bowler hat bobbing. There was nothing odd about a woman running through the fields. On this high plateau of Peru, near the shores of Lake Titicaca, for some reason, I discovered, people frequently break into a short-stepped trot; only visitors from the lowlands found it remarkable because here, at 12,600 feet (3,800 meters) above sea level, all extra effort is difficult and even painful. Oxygen starvation causes loss of appetite and inhibits sleep; even a short walk up a steep hill set my heart pounding and my lungs gasping for precious oxygen. And yet, I couldn't help but marvel at how the local people jog-trotted so cheerfully along, often with a bulky load on their backs, as if they could keep up their pace for hours on end.

What *was* odd, though, about Mrs. Andrea Curaci running to meet me and my interpreter, Graciela Laura de Almonte, in the summer of 1977, was that she hadn't been notified to expect us. The road we were on led to a big trout farm, visited by many cars and vans. Yet as she reached the forecourt of her little thatched home—in no way out of breath as we both were—she told us: "I knew you were coming today; that is why I came running."

Mrs. Curaci was in those days (she has since deceased) a *partera empirica*—a traditional midwife. This then 53-year-old healer was also a bonesetter, famed throughout her district for healing broken joints. She was a fortune-teller and a folk healer *extraordinaire*. But what was more important (and the reason for us being there), she had "second sight" and could see into the future. So Graciela and I let pass without comment her casual statement that she knew we were coming.

The black bowler with a tassel crowned a neat figure dressed in a dark blue jacket, a red skirt, and worn black slippers. Under the bowler hat her graying hair hung in pigtails. Pinned on to one shoulder was some stinging nettle. Through my interpreter I inquired as to the purpose of that and she responded that she had just got through treating three patients (two female and one male, all past fifty years of age) about an hour before we arrived. Their conditions were all the same, though the manifestations varied from patient to patient: They suffered from varying forms of mental derangement.

She claimed the nettle exerted a calming influence upon her as well as her patients, so that she could effectively treat them. She said that nettle was by far the best remedy she had ever found for mental illness. We went inside her little home with its straw roof and cracked mud-packed walls, which made one think of the legend of Hansel and Gretel, though our hostess was not at all witchlike.

She explained how she used a combination of prayer, lit candies, divination, and plenty of *warm* stinging nettle tea to help those in fear of losing their minds regain their confidence and have their sanity restored again.

Interestingly, most of those who came to her for treatment of their mental problems lived *lower down*. In other words, she observed for us, those who resided at the level she and her husband did seldom ever became depressed or experienced any type of mental breakdown. I attribute this to a lack of positive air ions and free radicals found so commonly in air pollution.

I gazed our the open door of her hut to the handful of mud-walled thatched cottages below. The hillside fell away to a little valley which opened on to the shore of Lake Titicaca, whose pastel blue waters stretched away in a northeasterly direction to where it seemed to touch the horizon. "You must be very happy to live in such a place as this," I told her through Graciela. Mrs. Curaci smiled, nodded her agreement, then said, "Yes, for it is here that the mind is free, the heart happy, and the spirit *always* overjoyed!"

OBESITY. "Which form of physical exercise do you think is the best to lose weight by?" When I put this question to folk healers from Indonesia, Afghanistan, Turkey, and Tibet, every one of them was of the same opinion that *walking* is by far "the simplest, cheapest, and most convenient way" to take off excess weight. But if the goal for someone is to lose weight, a mere easy stroll just won't cut it. The fact is, a 150-pound person burns less than 100 calories on a leisurely half-hour walk. (And weight-loss experts say that most Americans, Canadians, and Europeans who need to lose significant weight should decrease the calories they consume and increase the calories they burn by a total of at least 500 calories per day.)

But the folk healers I spoke with all felt that what it really took to lose meaningful weight was to turn up the intensity of a walk so more calories could be burned off. They gave several suggestions for how they thought this might be accomplished.

While strolling might have some health benefits, yet it is brisk walking—at a pace that makes it tough to talk, which means at least two miles in 30 minutes—that is guaranteed to help you shed more pounds. Walking fast allows you to cover more ground and work more muscles than merely walking slow. At a very quick pace, you'll burn almost as many calories as you do while jogging, with less stress on your body.

Form is important here; the right posture helps you move faster. Here's what to do: Walk tall and stay relaxed. Bend your elbows at 90-degree angles and keep them close to your body. Swing your arms forcefully so that your hands are level with your breastbone on the upswing and almost brush your hips on the downswing. Instead of lengthening your steps, keep your stride short and quick. Land on your heels and roll through your foot to push off firmly with your toes.

Remember this: If you walk at 3 mph for 30 minutes, you burn 119 calories; if you walk at 4.5 mph for 30 minutes, you burn 153 calories.

Invest more time in what you do. Most of us think that walking three times a week for 30 minutes at a time is the magic weight-off formula, but research has shown that's simply not enough. It was discovered that people who were successful at weight loss burned the number of calories that a person would by walking about an hour a day, nearly every day of the week.

If you're already walking three days a week, gradually build to six or seven days a week, my folk healer consultants suggested. At the same time, they insisted that a person should stretch his or her walks to 45 minutes or an hour. If this sounds overwhelming, bear in mind that you can get roughly the same benefits by splitting your walk into three or four 15-minute walks throughout the day.

And don't forget this: If you walk 30 minutes at 4 mph, you burn 136 calories, whereas if you walk 60 minutes at 4 mph, you burn 272 calories.

And try alternating between a brisk pace and short periods at an even faster pace. (You should still be able to speak, but only a few breathless words.) You'll not only increase your calorie burn, but also strengthen your cardiovascular system and become a faster walker over time.

There are basically two ways to begin. The easiest is the land-mark method. If you walk in your neighborhood, try changing your pace at every other stop sign or park bench. If you walk on a track, walk one speed on the straightaways and another on the curves. The other option is using a watch to time yourself. There should be 1 minute fast walking followed by 2 minutes moderate, gradually working up to 1 minute fast for every 1 minute moderate.

Oh, by the way, keep this in mind: If you walk 30 minutes at a moderate but continuous pace, you burn 136 calories, whereas if you walk 30 minutes, switching to a faster pace 15 times, you burn 146 calories.

Try walking up an incline or stairs whenever possible. This not only increases your caloric expenditure but also tones the muscles in your buttocks and thighs because it demands more from your legs. Find a natural hill or use the stairs in a local park or stadium. You can also use a treadmill and adjust the incline. To get the most calorie-burning benefits you want, you'll need to spend most of a 30-minute walk heading uphill. If your hill is small, you may need to climb it several times to achieve this result.

Because hill walking can be hard on your knees and lower back, it's important to use proper form. Lean slightly forward from your hips and shorten your stride; this gives you the extra power you need to tackle a hill. Going downhill is even harder on your body than going uphill, so take controlled steps. Again, lean slightly forward, decrease your stride, and keep your knees bent. For really steep hills, my folk healer informants recommended crisscrossing at an angle to reduce the strain on your muscles and joints.

SEXUALLY TRANSMITTED DISEASES. Folk healers throughout the Middle East declare in no uncertain terms that olive leaf (*Olea europaea*) is one of the very best plant remedies to treat even the most aggressive cases of sexually transmitted diseases (STDs). The antimicrobial agent in this leaf kills viruses, including the common cold, herpes, and Epstein-Barr, as well as bacteria that cause illnesses such as sinusitis and bronchitis.

Olive trees and shrubs grow in southern Europe and quite plentifully in the Mediterranean regions. The hills of Israel, Jordan, Iran, Iraq, and Syria are filled with millions of them. The olive tree, some say, is almost as old as the Bible itself, in terms of recorded historical usage.

The dried leaves contain the most important medicinal components of the herb. One of them is oleuropein, which is converted in the body in two types of elenoic acid. These acids interfere with the amino acid production necessary for those viruses and bacteria that cause STDs to thrive; this action prevents them from replicating.

Most of the studies of olive leaf extract have been done on oleuropein. One lab study published in 1993 in the *Journal of Applied Bacteriology* reported that a 2 percent concentration of oleuropein delayed the growth of *Staphylococcus aureus,* an infectious bacteria commonly spread in hospitals, by up to 30 hours; higher concentrations of oleuropein inhibited bacterial growth entirely. Syrian, Egyptian, and Israeli clinical studies have demonstrated that when the entire olive leaf itself is used, STDs are substantially reduced in number and their chances of recurrence also become very low.

Olive leaf extract is most effective when taken as a capsule standardized to 6 percent oleuropein. It is recommended that one 500-milligram capsule per day be taken to fight any existing bacterial or viral infections, especially those brought on by STDs. You can also obtain oleuropein—enough for prevention but not therapeutic doses—from olive leaf tea. Boil 2 teaspoons of crushed, dried leaves in 1 cup of water for 10 minutes; drink 4 cups daily.

TUBERCULOSIS.   A somewhat novel treatment for wind-related illnesses that include tuberculosis (TB), pneumonia, influenza, and the common cold exists among Cambodian, Laotian, and Vietnamese immigrants to the United States. It is coin rubbing and boiled coin tea. Strange though they are by our standards, both methods of coin therapy seem to work!

The lay practice of *cao gió* (as it is called in Vietnam) is quite commonly used among American Vietnamese for all respiratory ailments, including fever, chills, and headaches. A native folk healer who has immigrated to the United States from this Southeast Asian country will ask the patient to remove his shirt or her blouse, so that the skin is bare. Peanut or coconut oil is then liberally applied to the back and chest with cotton balls or swabs. The skin is massaged until warm. Firm downward strokes with the edge of a silver coin (half dollar or dollar) are used until purplish spots or patches appear.

An unfortunate cultural consequence of this relatively harmless folk remedy is that in some instances when such a thing has been performed on the back of a young child who is later admitted to a hospital for something else, the medical staff there may incorrectly interpret it to be some form of physical child abuse. This has happened a few times in the past where the admitted children showed evidence of dramatic purplish marks in linear patterns over the anterior and posterior trunks. Child services and the local police were promptly notified much to the consternation and confusion of parents and relatives who, in many cases, couldn't speak a word of English. However, when a translator was brought in and authorities were satisfied that it was simply an old-fashioned folk remedy, then the parents were released from police custody and their seized children given back to them.

Several silver coins (half-dollars or dollars) are boiled in a pint of hot water for 10 minutes. The tea is removed from the heat, covered, and allowed to steep for 30 minutes. One cup of this warm *colloidal* silver solution is taken every couple of hours. (It's advisable to scrub the coins well with soap and rinse them under cold water before using them to make a tea, considering how filthy money can get through the exchange of numerous hands.)

UNDERWEIGHT. My father's brother-in-law, a retired carpenter named Thomas Gordon Liddiard, died in the summer of 1993 at the age of 89. He was in and out of hospitals for the last 30 years of his life, suffering from a number of different ailments. In the last year or so of his existence, he lost a great deal of weight. The doctors didn't seem to know what to do to reverse this, which comes as no surprise seeing as how they get very little training in medical school in nutrition or dietetics.

One time I went to visit this man while he was a patient at LDS Hospital here in Salt Lake City. A young, former friend of mine by the name of Matt Fountaine accompanied me. Tom, then 88 years of age, lay in bed in apparently great pain. He hadn't slept a wink the night before and wanted the nurse to get him some sleeping pills so he could rest properly, but she claimed only the doctor could authorize this. Understandably, then, he was in a very cranky and ill-tempered mood when we stopped by to see him.

After seating ourselves and making some small talk with him, we both were surprised to see him grasp the railing on the side of his bed, pull himself up into a sitting position, and bellow out in a voice loud enough to be heard in that wing of the hospital: "You both need to understand something here. Let me give you a piece of good advice. You need to learn to be your own doctor! You need to learn how to take care of yourself, so you don't have to be in a place like this!" He momentarily paused long enough to lick his thin, dry lips, before continuing on: "By gawd! It's so miserable here! I feel like I'm in some sort of hell. Just look at me, will you?"

With that he savagely pulled up his hospital gown almost to his chest, revealing an emaciated frame of nothing but skin and bones that had once been a lean and muscular physique. "Look what they've done to me! By gawd! They're starving me to death. I eat and eat every thing they bring me and then ask for more, but am denied extra food. 'Hospital policy,' they tell me. 'Sorry, but we can't give you another meal unless the doctors on duty order it.' I'm sick of it, just plain sick of it, I tell you." Then leaning over on his left side, he shook a bony finger in both our faces and declared in understandable wrath, "Don't ever let yourselves get into a place like this, if you can [at all] avoid it!" (Mr. Liddiard had been hospitalized for a week for pneumonia, which was successfully treated with drugs; but ironically enough, he suffered from hospital-induced malnourishment and died from *starvation!*)

Following this unhappy and troubling episode, I began an earnest quest for those things which would prevent something like this from ever happening to anyone that I knew who was elderly and had to be hospitalized for some reason. Those items I found which can prevent unnecessary weight loss during recuperation from an illness are as follows: soy milk and soy powder shakes; slippery elm bark powder in the form of a warm gruel or mush, or slippery elm bark powder capsules; fenugreek seed tea; and Tocomin brand tocotrienol complex, a very innovative vitamin E for the twenty-first century from Malaysia.

Soybean has been recognized for a long time now as being a very useful and nutritive food; its inclusion in the diet in the form of soy milk or soy shakes will not only provide nourishment but also help prevent tissue wasting. Slippery elm inner bark and fenugreek seed are quite mucilaginous (slimy) substances which promote digestion, build strength, and contribute to tissue mass. Tocomin, a palm-derived vitamin E sold exclusively by Carotech, Inc., stabilizes muscle and nerve tissue and prevents their shrinkage during periods of long convalescence. (See the Appendix for more information concerning some of the items mentioned here.)

In addition to the things just given, there are also other weight-gaining foods to be considered: nuts, nut butters, seeds and seed oils, okra (especially in the form of gumbo), and root vegetables such as potatoes, yams, sweet potatoes, carrots, parsnips, turnips, and rutabagas. Where such foods, herbs, and supplements have been consistently used by the elderly before, during, and after hospitalization, there has been very *little* loss of weight; none of those who've followed this program ever suffered from underweight or died of miserable starvation as Tom Liddiard did.

WORMS.   The best herbal tonic for getting rid of intestinal parasites and worms of any description is made in Calgary, Canada, by Flora Beverage Co. Ltd. and is marketed under the name of Essex Botanical. It includes purified water, burdock root, sheep sorrel, slippery elm bark, and rhubarb root. The formula was originally developed by an old Ojibway Indian shaman in the Province of Ontario many years ago, thoroughly tested and improved upon by a Canadian nurse, and finally manufactured on a large scale in the proper way it should have been by a Hungarian businessman.

Essex is a classic example of something wonderful that happens when a particular remedy receives the benefits of what I call "cultural blending." In this case, three distinct cultures were involved in its present state: Native American, Canadian, and Hungarian. Each person made his or her own contribution to this formula and the world at large now benefits from their combined but distinct inputs.

Essex is completely safe and may be given to young or old alike without any problems. It is a general tonic for the whole body, providing strength and stamina for even the weakest physical systems when used on a regular basis. (See the Appendix for more information.)

Real Folk Medicine

Through the many years of research into just about every corner of the globe, I've come to discern as a medical anthropologist what I believe to be genuine folk medicine. It isn't always the kind practiced by alternative doctors or chiropractors in sterile clinics. Nor is it the distribution of herbal products and nutritional supplements through health food stores and networking (multilevel) companies.

Rather it is the simple treatment of disease by unlicensed and often poorly educated practitioners using primitive remedies and intuitive skills endowed them by a Supreme Being or Supreme Power in whom they usually manifest implicit confidence as they're guided in what they are doing. And their customary payments for such folk medical services may be squawking chickens, pieces of cooked pork, fresh fruit and vegetables, eggs, milk, cheese, butter, coffee, beans, soda pop, or sometimes even money.

These men and women often devote their entire lives to the care of others, taking very little for themselves and nearly always ascribing the successes of their remarkable healing abilities to something or

Someone higher than themselves. Always humble, generally honest, and forever compassionate, they see sick people night and day, in rain or shine, whether convenient or inconvenient to their schedules.

Such a one was Doña Ascensión Solórsano, the very last San Juan Indian of Gilroy, California, who died long before I was born. But her remedies and the unique culture from which she came were faithfully preserved on record by ethnologist John P. Harrington for the world to enjoy shortly before she died. She is the one to whom this book has been dedicated; and if you haven't yet read my dedication to her at the front of this book, then may I suggest you do so in order to become better acquainted with this sweet soul of a woman.

Another such dear soul was my own sainted Grandmother Barbara Liebhardt Heinerman, who herself in many ways paralleled the uncontained goodness that the former did. And when she passed on at an incredibly advanced age, she left not only a written record of her work, but also a visual and spoken memory with one of her two grandsons, namely myself. And like Harrington of the Smithsonian Institution, this anthropologist in the later years of his life has endeavored to publicize some of his grandmother's own healing remedies as well.

But beyond what she left behind, Grandmother Barbara also imparted to me, *while still alive,* "a healer's intuition" in my early childhood. This, I consider to be, the single, *greatest gift* of all, for it has enabled me to bless mankind with folk medical wisdom in the same way that she did and all of those who preceded her.

This is the fine tradition that anyone who has ever been, now is, or will yet become a true and caring folk healer eventually inherits and passes on to the next generation. I believe that with this book I have done just that for those who will follow after me. God bless them and everyone who entrust their health and well-being to men and women of such high caliber like this.

Appendix

This section provides information for those who may wish to contact a specific individual or organization regarding particular remedies, herbs or supplements mentioned in this book. The author has no financial interest in these organizations but simply mentions them and their products as a service to readers.

NATURALLY VITAMINS
4404 East Elwood
Phoenix, AZ 85040
800-899-4499
Fax: 480-991-0551
E-mail: info@naturallyvitamins.com

Exclusive distributors of the world-renowned Wobenzym N product. The company offers a complete line of nutritional supplements for optimal health and well-being. With European ownership and German technology, it produces effective vitamin/mineral products that are unbeatable.

EARTH'S PHARMACY
131 West 500 South
PMB #422
Bountiful, UT 84010
800-676-4898
Fax: 801-451-2306
Website: http://www.earthspharmacy.com

The finest botanical line available anywhere in North America. State-of-the-art technology, top-quality materials, affordable prices, and people of integrity make this the one place to do all of your herbal shopping via the Internet, by telephone, or through mail-order.

CAROTECH INC
21 Balmoral Court
Talmadge Village
Edison, NJ 08817
732-906-1901
Fax: 732-906-1902
Website: www.tocotrienol.org.

This company, with headquarters in Malaysia, is the world's only technologically integrated plant capable of extracting tocotrienols complex, mixed carotene, and phytosterols from the palm fruits. Tocomin is their flagship vitamin E product for the new millennium.

FLORA BEVERAGE CO. LTD.
Bay "F," 2828-54th Avenue SE
Calgary, Alberta, Canada T2C 0A7
403-236-0155
Fax: 403-236-0155

This company is the exclusive manufacturer for the world-famous Essex Botanical, and other equally fine Canadian herbal bitters for complete gastrointestinal health and total physical rejuvenation.

TIANSHI HEALTH PRODUCTS, INC.
728-134th Street, SW, Suite 222
Everett, WA 98204
425-741-2289
Fax: 425-741-8728
Website: www.tianshiusa.com

Originally founded in the People's Republic of China by Li Jinyuan seven years ago, this remarkable health supplements company now has locations in more than a dozen countries around the world. With more than six million distributors of its many excellent products, it is the largest of its kind on earth. The Chinese formulations it markets are based on 4,000 years of empirical use and historical authenticity. They are the best Chinese traditional medicines to be found anywhere.

WAKUNAGA OF AMERICA CO. LTD.
23501 Madero
Mission Viejo, CA 92691-2744
949-855-2776
Fax: 949-587-5053
Website: www.kyolic.com

This is the American marketing arm for the parent company of Hiroshima, Japan, Wakunaga Pharmaceutical Co. Using German ingenuity and Japanese technological know-how, the world's first and only aged garlic extract was developed and perfected. Currently solid worldwide under the brand name of Kyolic, this one-of-a-kind garlic product has proven to be more effective than any of its numerous competitors. It also has the unique distinction of being the most scientifically studied commercial garlic product in the world.

PINES INTERNATIONAL
P. O. Box 1107
Lawrence, KS 66044
800-MY PINES (800-697-4637)

This is the maker of extraordinary chlorophyll products that include wheat grass powder, barley grass powder, and a multiple cereal grasses-and-herbal-complex known as Mighty Greens. It also makes and distributes the nation's only organic beet juice concentrate powder. The company is one of the very few Anglo-owned nutritional companies which contributes a portion of its annual corporate profits to support worthy Native American causes.

In addition,

JOHN HEINERMAN, Folk Healer
P. 0. Box 11471
Salt Lake City, UT 84147
801-521-8824

The author of this work will gladly assist you any way he can and makes himself available for this purpose.